Privileges of Birth

Fertility, Reproduction and Sexuality

General Editors:

Soraya Tremayne, Founding Director, Fertility and Reproduction Studies Group and Research Associate, Institute of Social and Cultural Anthropology, University of Oxford.

Marcia C. Inhorn, William K. Lanman, Jr. Professor of Anthropology and International Affairs, Yale University.

Philip Kreager, Director, Fertility and Reproduction Studies Group, and Research Associate, Institute of Social and Cultural Anthropology and Institute of Human Sciences, University of Oxford.

Understanding the complex and multifaceted issue of human reproduction has been, and remains, of great interest both to academics and practitioners. This series includes studies by specialists in the field of social, cultural, medical and biological anthropology, medical demography, psychology and development studies. Current debates and issues of global relevance on the changing dynamics of fertility, human reproduction and sexuality are addressed.

Recent volumes:

Volume 44
Privileges of Birth: Constellations of Care, Myth and Race in South Africa
Jennifer J.M. Rogerson

Volume 43
Access to Assisted Reproductive Technologies: The Case of France and Belgium
Edited by Jennifer Merchant

Volume 42
Making Bodies Kosher: The Politics of Reproduction among Haredi Jews in England
Ben Kasstan

Volume 41
Elite Malay Polygamy: Wives, Wealth and Woes in Malaysia
Miriam Koktvedgaard Zeitzen

Volume 40
Being a Sperm Donor: Masculinity, Sexuality, and Biosociality in Denmark
Sebastian Mohr

Volume 39
Global Fluids: The Cultural Politics of Reproductive Waste and Value
Charlotte Kroløkke

Volume 38
Reconceiving Muslim Men: Love and Marriage, Family and Care in Precarious Times
Edited by Marcia C. Inhorn and Nefissa Naguib

Volume 37
The Anthropology of the Fetus: Biology, Culture, and Society
Edited by Sallie Han, Tracy K. Betsinger, and Amy K. Scott

Volume 36
Fertility, Conjuncture, Difference: Anthropological Approaches to the Heterogeneity of Modern Fertility Declines
Edited by Philip Kreager and Astrid Bochow

Volume 35
The Online World of Surrogacy
Zsuzsa Berend

For a full volume listing, please see the series page on our website: http://www.berghahnbooks.com/series/fertility-reproduction-and-sexuality

PRIVILEGES OF BIRTH
Constellations of Care, Myth and Race in South Africa

Jennifer J.M. Rogerson

berghahn
NEW YORK • OXFORD
www.berghahnbooks.com

First published in 2020 by

Berghahn Books

www.berghahnbooks.com

Library of Congress Cataloging-in-Publication Data

Names: Rogerson, Jennifer J. M., author.
Title: Privileges of birth : constellations of care, myth and race in South Africa / Jennifer J. M. Rogerson.
Other titles: Fertility, reproduction, and sexuality ; v. 44.
Description: New York : Berghahn Books, 2020. | Series: Fertility, reproduction and sexuality: social and cultural perspectives; volume 44 | Includes bibliographical references and index.
Identifiers: LCCN 2019038003 (print) | LCCN 2019038004 (ebook) | ISBN 9781789204353 (hardback) | ISBN 9781789204360 (ebook)
Subjects: LCSH: Childbirth--Social aspects--South Africa. | Midwifery--South Africa. | Postnatal care--Social aspects--South Africa. | Maternal health services--South Africa. | Newborn infants--Care--Social aspects--South Africa.
Classification: LCC RG652 .R64 2020 (print) | LCC RG652 (ebook) | DDC 362.198400968--dc23
LC record available at https://lccn.loc.gov/2019038003
LC ebook record available at https://lccn.loc.gov/2019038004

British Library Cataloguing in Publication Data

A catalogue record for this book is available from the British Library

ISBN 978-1-78920-435-3 hardback
ISBN 978-1-78920-436-0 ebook

Contents

Introduction. Elite Birthing Care in South Africa 1

Chapter 1. Myths of Birth: Intervention, Having 'Choice' and Histories of Birth 25

Chapter 2. Being Heard: Planning, 'Choice' and Knowing in Pregnancy and Birth 58

Chapter 3. Self-Making: Pain, Language and Metaphor in Birth Stories 97

Chapter 4. Making Birthing Relations: The Constitution of Attentiveness and Responsiveness 133

Conclusion. Care as a Problem, Care's Limits 164

Appendix 169

Glossary 170

References 175

Index 191

Introduction

Elite Birthing Care in South Africa

The floor to ceiling wall made entirely of glass offered a clear, expansive view of the ocean. The living room was open-plan, and bright as light streamed in through the glass walls and ceiling. The dining table, with a fresh flower centrepiece, was contemporary and surrounded by Scandinavian modern chairs, scattered with sheepskins, a fashion in 2015. Sandy, as I call her, welcomed me into her home, offering me filtered water infused with cucumber; she showed me where her private, one-to-one Hypnobirthing classes were going to take place in the living room. She explained that her husband travelled for work much of the time and fitting in birthing classes was easier if these took place in their home, at a time that suited the couple. Participating in Hypnobirthing classes was a common activity for women using private midwives; they understood the classes as a method that would help facilitate the 'natural' births they desired.

Sandy's home and her aspirations are typical of the circumstances and birthing desires of women using private midwives who I would come to know and observe over my year in the midwives' practices. Yet these women and their socio-economic contexts are atypical in South Africa. The group of women with whom I worked are unusual in South Africa's birthing sector for two reasons. The first reason is that they are able to access private health care, a form of care that is only available to South Africa's (largely white) financially elite class. This means that they are able to 'choose' how to birth. The second reason these women are unusual is that even though they would be birthing using private birthing services, they hoped for 'natural births'. This is uncommon in South Africa's private sector as most women able to access private health care birth via caesarean section (C-section).

This is an ethnography about the constellation of care, race and privilege as they materialise in middle-class women's birthing practices. It traces privilege as choice, privilege as isolation, privilege and capital, and privilege and race as these emerge in relation to recognition and care. Care and being able to make choices about it form the central themes running through the book. This, in a South African setting with State health services under strain, understaffed and underequipped, is not a given but a kind of entitlement and an option for only a few. This is because South Africa's medical care is divided between private and public sectors. Where and how one births is largely determined by the sector a woman is able to access.

Birthing in South Africa

Rachel and I sat in her home in Somerset West, a small town on the outskirts of Cape Town, three weeks after the birth of her son. It was still chilly in the early days of spring but it was sunny so we sat near the window and Rachel spent most of her time speaking with me, breastfeeding or holding her baby. Rachel told me how she had gone into labour three weeks early and the speed of events had caught her and her husband, Dan, off guard. She had still been working (indeed she believed her annoyance at a work situation had contributed to the early onset of her labour) but was now completely focused on her baby, commenting on how she could not believe how she had made work such a priority before the arrival of her son. Rachel described her experiences and reasons for choosing a midwife-led birth. She explained what her friend had said:

> My friend, Dina, she's one of the smallest woman I've ever met and she had all three of her children naturally. She said you have to find the right practitioner that believes in the *power of a woman's body.* She said that's what you need to do and stay away from paternalistic men who believe it's unnatural and that they are doing you and your husband a favour by cutting the baby out of you cos you're going to be so damaged afterwards.

This was a common theme amongst my informants. Strong views on birthing highlight ideas of paternalism and feminism in my study. The overlaps on opinions of birth are also significant: I will explore these themes. How such opinions emerged is framed within South Africa's approach to health care.

Private Sector Settings and Defining the Middle Class

There are two means of accessing medical care in South Africa: private and public sector led care services. Women with medical aid or enough money to pay out-of-pocket who are therefore able to use private care have the 'option' of how they give birth. Private care obstetricians offer vaginal birth and elective C-sections (and emergency C-sections) and medical aid covers the costs of a C-section more readily than a midwife-led vaginal birth (Macdonald 2008). Despite the fact that birth is unpredictable, women using private medical care are able to plan and think around how they birth as a choice-based practice.

As a woman living in Cape Town, South Africa, Rachel was included in a socio-economic bracket that allowed her to pay for monthly medical aid cover and she accessed private health care. The majority of the women in my study had medical aid and were either working or had partners who earned enough money so that they were able to not work and could afford private care as a family unit under their partner's medical aid scheme.[1] I refer to these women as middle-class but the definition and criteria for a middle-class population is complex. Visagie and Posel (2011) argue that South Africa's middle class is hard to define. Being middle class may be classified as having reached a particular level of affluence and lifestyle. It can also be defined on a comparative basis, relative to the economic position of other members of a population. A middle income in relation to the general populous is not adequate in South Africa where the average middle income places people at or just below the poverty line. Using criteria of affluence and lifestyle, such as being able to afford private health care, having housekeeping services (caring for children and household), owning a car and having tertiary education provides a means of defining women in my study as middle-class that is congruent with definitions in developed countries.[2] Having said that, while women in this study mainly had to work in order to maintain their lifestyles, the gap between the rich and poor in South Africa is enormous; inequality is still largely racially stratified, and South Africa remains one of the most unequal countries in the world in terms of income distribution.[3]

The women with whom I worked in this research subjectively defined themselves as middle-class and fell into categories of being middle-class in terms of the definition offered above, but the care they were able to access and their lifestyles, by the standards of the majority of South Africans, were elite. My study thus concerns an elite version of formal care, the meaning of care in this context and how women accessed and navigated particular versions of birth and care. As I will show, where and how one accesses care in South Africa determines how one is cared for. The elite quality of care is significant.

Rachel had access to various options of care and intended to birth in a private medical institution but she faced challenges in opting to birth 'naturally' (that is, vaginally) as this meant finding a health care provider who was willing and able to offer support for a vaginal birth.[4] While this may seem simple, 72 per cent of women in South Africa's private sector birth via C-section, with some private hospitals reporting C-section rates of 90 per cent (Fokazi 2011, Smith 2014). The World Health Organization (WHO)has stated that C-section rates should be between 10 and 15 per cent in any country, and in the light of new research on the benefits of vaginal delivery to infants, WHO states that vaginal birth should be the way that most women birth.

Patients using private sector medical services in South Africa have become more litigious. Obstetricians pay approximately R40 000 (about $3500) per month on medical malpractice insurance as more legal cases have emerged with adverse birth outcomes (Roux and van Rensburg 2011). Women are given the 'choice' of how they birth and the statistics suggest that many choose to have an elective C-section. Concurrently, higher monthly costs for doctors mean that obstetricians fit in more deliveries via C-section, where allotted times and days are set, and surgery takes less time than assisting labouring women over hours, potentially through the night (Fokazi 2011). The merging of financial imperatives, convenience, medical aid willing to cover C-sections more readily than midwife-led care home or hospital based births (although more providers of medical aid are becoming willing to cover midwife-attended birth) (MacDonald 2008) contributes to high C-section numbers. The midwives in my study established themselves as the caring alternative to obstetric-led birth which was criticised for scaring women and overriding patient decision-making. These factors, together with the desire for C-sections by many South African women, have produced the high C-section statistics in South

Africa's private sector (Fokazi 2011). Indeed, WHO released a statement on the rise in C-section rates globally and in all health care sectors (WHO 2015). WHO has reviewed the data and finds no benefit from a C-section birth to women or baby at the population level of rates higher than 10 per cent.[5]

The rising global C-section rates and high C-section rates in South Africa's private sector are not the only concern for pregnant women accessing private care. Women in the private sector reported not getting ideal care and being forced into C-sections when they did not believe they needed one (Roux and van Rensburg 2011). Concomitantly, women in the public sector also report inadequate care (Vivian et al. 2011, Jewkes et al. 1998). The question of what defines adequate and inadequate care is apposite. In both sectors of medical care there have been reports of inadequate care but it is mainly middle-class women who use the private sector and largely working-class women who receive public sector care. The public sector provides care for 82 per cent of South Africa's population but only accounts for 40 per cent of health expenditure in South Africa. There is a wide gap between care and resources in the different health care sectors (Pillay 2009). The question of whether definitions of adequacy in care differ by class warrants attention. My study focuses on a version of care available largely to middle-class women; therefore, care and its adequacy across sectors is important.

The Western Cape Government website on maternal and women's health offers a description of birth/labour services. The website recommends that labouring women bring a birthing partner (partner, friend or doula) to accompany them during labour. A birthing partner is encouraged as the website states that women feel more supported and need less pain medication (indeed epidurals are not an option in Midwife Obstetric Units [MOUs] where low-risk births in the public sector occur). In public sector birthing venues, mainly MOUs, midwives work on shifts and labour care consists of checking the progress of labour and monitoring the wellness of women and babies. Continuous, one-to-one labour care is not offered as there are not enough midwives on duty to support the number of labouring women individually each day. Conditions in public sector hospitals are difficult. Staff are overburdened and Vivian et al. (2011) and Jewkes et al. (1998) report patient abuse. Overburdened midwives and nursing personnel were reported to have shouted at labouring women and scolded young unmarried women for being pregnant. Adequate care in the public sector context was defined as women receiving care that facilitated healthy women and babies, 'adequate' stay time in hospital (six or more hours) and no patient abuse (Jewkes et al. 1998). By contrast, the women in my study saw adequacy of care as predicated on continued close attention and extended interpersonal relations between women and carers over time, rather than on whether or not they survived childbirth and delivered live babies.

Women using private care defined adequate care on a spectrum of quality of care and continuity thereof because they were approaching care as consumers. Women in private care were given rest-in periods in hospital as medical aid covers the cost of a hospital stay for three days for a vaginal birth and up to five days for a C-section (women who birth in MOUs in contrast are given a few hours to rest as there are not enough hospital beds for longer rest-in periods). Women in my study had private rooms but reported a lack of one-to-one care while in labour as obstetricians mainly only assist women and enter the labour room at the second stage of labour (delivery). Particular expectations of care and accompaniment held by different groups of women define the parameters of adequate care and differentiate conceptualisations of 'adequate care' for various classes of South Africa's population. It is important therefore, to explore what care means in specific contexts. It also makes space for examining care in relation to race and privilege.

Accessing Independent Midwifery Care

Desiring a vaginal birth and a particular version of care rather than an obstetric-led birth that she believed could easily lead to a C-section, Rachel looked to a small number of independent midwives operating in nearby suburbs who were willing to support what she understood to be her choice of a 'natural' birth. At the time of my research, there were eight independent midwives working in the leafy middle-class suburbs of Cape Town, providing women with midwife-led care and offering vaginal, 'intervention-free' 'natural' birth where possible. Seven of these eight midwives and their clients are the focus of my work. The midwives in the study had been in private practice for between fifteen and twenty years, building a reputation for offering desired versions of birth ('natural birth') in the context of rising C-section rates in the private sector in Cape Town. Even though the midwives were all biomedically trained and relied on obstetric back-up and medicalised versions of safe practice, they explicitly contrasted their work with what they described as technocratic/obstetric models of birth. Indeed, the team midwives (explained below) in my study had a C-section rate of 17 per cent.[6]

Midwives in South Africa were part of and were influenced by broader international debates on birth. Like the United States-based Midwifery Model of Care™ (MMC), they set their model of birth against medicalised versions of birth, particularly those that involved surgical intervention or medication. The midwives worked from the perspective that birth is normal and natural and that too much 'unnecessary' intervention is detrimental to a pregnant woman and her baby. Yet these versions of birth and the associated training of professionals were not all that different from one another. There were also overlaps in training depending on which sector of care one used.

Overlaps between Private and Public Sector Settings

The birthing context in South Africa is highly medicalised. Most births occur in a medical facility, and 84.4 per cent of women have a skilled attendant assisting at their delivery (Tlebere et al. 2007). South Africa is in fact well provided in terms of obstetric care. There are six basic essential (defined as providing sufficient medical care for low-risk women and births) obstetric care facilities per 500,000 people (well above the recommended rate internationally of four per 500,000 people). Despite this, there are challenges to birthing (Tlebere et al. 2007). South Africa has committed to the Sustainable Development Goals (SDG). These include reducing the maternal mortality rate to 38 per 100,000 live births and the infant mortality rate to 18 per 1000 live births.

Given that half of women in developing countries do not get the health care they need, SDG goals include improving maternity care. Strategies to implement such goals include improving access to skilled birth attendants via dedicated obstetric ambulances and maternity waiting homes. In 2015 maternal mortality had been reduced to 138 per 100,000 live births but infant mortality is still high (World Bank 2015). While these numbers are contested due to underreporting and misclassification, there is general agreement that there is still work to be done in preventing maternal deaths in South Africa, and Bradshaw and Dorrington (2012) indicate that the maternal mortality rate is increasing despite the fact that 92 per cent of women receive antenatal care (WHO 2015, Bradshaw and Dorrington 2012). Strategies to improve these rates include access to immunisation, nutrition, increased maternal care, antenatal classes, encouraging breastfeeding, parenting classes and Kangaroo Mother Care, amongst others (Berry et al. 2013, Tshwane Declaration of support for breastfeeding 2011).

Public sector obstetrics care is provided through Midwife Obstetrics Units (MOUs) for low-risk births. These are staffed by public sector midwives. Training includes degree and diploma training. Both options consist of theoretical biomedical learning with a practical component taking place in hospitals throughout the four-year training period, providing clinical experience. Should the training for low-risk birth be insufficient due to complications in pregnancy, women are referred to second- and third-tier hospitals, depending on the severity of the complication(s). Unlike in the private sector, where women may use an array of specialists, including obstetricians/gynaecologists, general practitioners, independent midwives (and sometimes doulas) or another combination of carers, women in public sector care are usually attended to by nurses and midwives. As such, like the private sector, the kinds of care and levels of medicalisation available can vary widely depending on the level of health care tier and how high or low risk a pregnancy might be.

While independent midwives and public sector midwives working in MOUs are all registered with the South African Nursing Council as nurses/midwives, and have the same biomedical training, private sector midwives with whom I have worked made use of a particular model of care, The Midwives Model of Care™ (MMC). Monitoring the physical, psychological and social wellbeing of women and minimising surgical intervention are the benchmarks of this care model, a model that is not explicitly used in the state sector. Indeed, Chadwick et al. (2014) suggest that it is not implicit in public sector practice either. Midwives working in the public sector experience high volumes of labouring women without enough staff to offer continuous, one-on-one labour care. Vivian et al. (2011) described the abuses by midwives witnessed in a time pressured, overburdened public sector. Similarly trained but with different sets of concerns and challenges, independent midwives used the MMC in their practice.

According to Chadwick et al. (2014), difficulties faced in the public sector include a low standard of care, poor communication between care-givers and patients, and poor interpersonal treatment in maternity care (see also Jewkes et al. 1998). Heavy workloads and institutional stressors were acknowledged as reasons behind maternity service challenges (Penn-Kekana et al. 2007). Abrahams et al. (2001) report that in a study on maternal service provision in the Cape, pregnant women described being 'scolded' for presenting 'late' at clinics and felt dismissed and unheard by staff (see Ferreira 2016 for an account of 'lateness'). 'Abuse' and 'neglect' were commonly used to describe experiences at maternity clinics (Chadwick et al. 2014, Jewkes et al. 1998, Fonn et al. 1998, Vivian et al. 2011). Due to service and institutional difficulties (heavy workload, a high number of women requiring care from a limited number of care-givers, interpersonal and communication challenges), the MMC is not practised by public sector midwives.

Although the same professions and institutions are used by women in the public and private health sectors, the form of care instantiated by the MMC and independent midwives is available mainly to middle-class women and their partners through private health care provision where medical aid that cover midwife-led birth pays for this service or women with medical aid that does not cover this version of care pay out-of-pocket. All of the midwives participating in my study of private midwife-attended birth offered home births and hospital births. Despite being part of the private sector of health care provision, almost all the midwives offered hospital births at both a private and a public hospital. This complicated and problematised the distinctions between public and private midwives and the care models used in institutions. Women who could afford an independent midwife could receive care practices based on the MMC but could birth their babies at a public hospital. Women using public sector care may birth their babies at the same hospital but receive a different kind of care even though their birth was being facilitated by someone of the same profession and in the same institution. Likewise, care within the public sector can also be highly varied. This blurs the boundaries, practices and definitions of institutions, institutional care and professions and raises the question of how care is constituted. I offer an ethnography of what I call 'a care world'. Thinking through care as a world draws attention to the multiple ways and factors that come to act on how care and care relations are made. It also places emphasis on the ways in which both carers and care-receivers actively produce care.

Elite Care, Race, Privilege and Apartheid

The women with whom I worked approached their births with particular ideas of birthing and choice that I explore throughout the chapters of this book. That they were able to approach birthing as a choice is shaped by race and racialised histories that come to bear on health care and its availability.

All aspects of South Africa's political, economic and social life are strongly linked to and moulded by its racialised beginnings, when white settlers began arriving in 1652, marking the beginnings of colonialism. South Africa was ruled as a colony, by the Dutch and later by the British, for almost 300 years before the solidification of institutionalised racial segregation of Apartheid in 1948. Apartheid was based on eugenic discourse and inherited colonial British laws, including those that separated non-white people from white people, and laws that required black people to travel with 'passes' when entering 'white areas'. Access to hospitals and medical care was segregated along racial lines. The availability of health care providers was also racially stratified. Therefore, South Africa's racialised nineteenth- and twentieth-century history (I explore this history more deeply in Chapter 1) produced a gendered, race-based stratification of birth attendants where the rural became conflated with women, lack of knowledge, lack of 'good care' and 'blackness' while civility, medical intervention, medical knowledge, 'whiteness' and men became the markers of urban, hospital-based birthing. Not only then were black people unable to access certain versions of care and facilities, but certain kinds of medical knowledge and care were conflated with race. I explore this theme in Chapter 1.

After years of discrimination, structural and physical violence and brutality, in 1994 Apartheid officially came to an end with the advent of the first democratic elections. The socio-economic effects still reverberate some twenty years later through all aspects of South African social life. Not only are economic inequalities still deeply entrenched; the devastating separation of people and discrimination towards black people have meant that the aspiration for an 'ordinary' suburban life is one that most South Africans are still unable to access (Ross 2010; see Burman and Reynolds 1986, Cock 1980 and May 2000 for a history of Apartheid and its consequences). Access to private health facilities and care is not available to most people. Yet, for many white South Africans, owning a home made of bricks and mortar, sending children to good schools and accessing private care is taken for granted. The disparities between the rich and the poor, the white and black population, in South Africa remain deeply stratified. Many white South Africans are able to take their life worlds for granted, as a group for whom liberal democracy works. Yet the lives of most of the women in my study are ones of great privilege. Specific conflations of whiteness and biomedicine on one side and blackness and 'local, lay' knowledge on the other are presently not as clear cut as the historical stratifications, but perceptions of how one births are attached to 'unruliness' and lack of biomedical facilities, and civility is conflated with technology. Who does caring and how is therefore apposite to questions of privilege.

This book focuses on one aspect of privilege: the access of private birthing care and, therefore, the availability of a series of affects. Tracing the constitution of care, the chapters articulate the different ways in which women using private midwifery care come to seek recognition for enacting work they regard as part of the 'universal feminine' in relation to reproduction. Thus, themes centre on birthing practices and reproduction. As I have shown, the specific version of care I focus on is available only to a small group of women in South Africa. Therefore, as I describe the ways in which women plan their births, engage with pain, and expect a certain kind of care, they become part of a birthing model in South Africa that reproduces privilege. The book articulates how the reproduction of privilege instantiates the reproduction of race in a South Africa where resources are still largely accessed by white people. Care, the ethics of care, resources and being able to make choices about these are themes to which I draw attention.

Framing and Theorising Care

My work offers an account of care, a subject to which anthropology has recently turned its attention. Indeed, the ethics of care come to inform and expand (as a set of ethics that are practised) within the models and modes of life that edify the ways in which pregnant women in my study wanted to be cared for. I look closely at the practices of care and how care is made (as a practise): this is broadly framed within a conversation with the ethics of care, offering an ethnographic account (see Tronto 1989, 1993, 2005, Sevenhuijsen 1998, 2000, 2003, Han 2012, Ticktin 2011 and Torres 2015 for the ethics and anthropology of care). Care as a practice – one of the elements that defines the ethics of care – is carefully examined, making care and its relation to the ethics of care an important aspect of this book. I examine how people access (via resources, language and myth) and co-produce their desired care, and how carers respond to care needs, arguing that the ways in which people desire and call for care – as a mode of recognition – is as much a part of the care dyad as are the care-giver's roles. I pay careful attention to the negotiated relationships that unfold in the client-midwife relationship and how these are shaped by and come to play out in the face of the models and myths that informed how women approached birth. I therefore draw attention to the ways in which care is part of broader influences (in this case birthing models, history and privilege) and how people constitute care in varied ways. Women wished to be seen as doing what they considered 'universally feminine work'; how they were cared for became part of how that work and birthing was understood. It also becomes one of the ways that privilege, and therefore race, is reproduced.

Getting to Know Midwives and Their Clients

When I began fieldwork in the spring of 2014, I worked with three midwives who were in private, single midwife practice (Alex, Alison and Bridget), as well as one team of midwives, The Cape Town Midwives, consisting of four midwives (Beth, Ingrid, Maggie and Tanya) who worked on a rotation basis of being 'on' and 'off' call, 'second on call', doing postnatal checks and antenatal consultations.[7] All the midwives had worked in public health at large teaching hospitals before moving to private care. The team versus single midwife approach was often spoken about because some pregnant women specifically chose their midwifery practice based on whether they would receive care throughout from one person or a team. For some women having a relationship with a single midwife was important as they felt they got to know her much better and believed that this was critical to the trust that they envisaged as being central to the birthing relationship they desired. For other women it was less important and they felt better knowing that there would always be a midwife available even if another women was in labour and they would get a 'fresh' midwife, not someone going to one labour straight after another labour (even though this was rare because 'single' midwives only took on four to six clients per month). The team approach meant women saw a different midwife at each consultation so that they had met and seen each midwife at least twice before going into labour, but they did not know who would be on call on their labour day. The team midwives spoke about not getting to know women as well as when they were in single midwife practice but not always being on call made life more manageable, and it meant they could care for more women.

On Method

I worked in the midwifery clinics for a year, tracking closely the activities of seven midwives and their clients. I interviewed nineteen women over the course of their pregnancies. Of these, I met six regularly both during their pregnancies and after the births and so we were able to become comfortable speaking with one another, often talking about matters unrelated to pregnancy and birth. I gained insight into how they lived and, for those wanting home births, how and where they imagined birthing. As partners or older siblings came and went during our conversations, the daily experiences, nuances and chaos of life were animated. Rather than just asking direct questions about birth, I was given a small window onto these women's life worlds and the influences and processes that enfleshed their crafting and imagining of birth as a plan. Sometimes I sat on the floor while a woman breastfed in the nursery where there was only one chair, or women bounced up and down on physiotherapy balls, trying to get their baby into a 'good position' for birth as we spoke. At other times, siblings woke from naps or came home from school so the children and I had brief 'chats', some children being curious about the new person in their home. During postnatal visits, the new baby was given to me to hold while women attended to something and I became officially acquainted with the little person who I had seen grow via their mothers' expanding bellies over several months.

As well as interviewing these women, I sat in on consultations with their midwives. With permission from midwives and clients, I attended almost 800 consultations between August 2014 and August 2015, providing the project with rich observational data. The booking appointment was the first consultation in a client's care trajectory. Here, midwives got to know their clients, conducting a thorough 'history-taking' and doing blood tests. Starting between 8:30am and 8:45am and running through until after lunch (approximately 2:30pm), midwives saw between five and eight women per day, with a few catch-up breaks between consultations as most of the midwives tended to spend longer with clients than scheduled.

I sat in the corner of the room during consultations so as not to be in women's lines of sight but women did often address me, asking for more details on the research. The women using the team midwives, whom I had seen each week in the last month of their pregnancy, would sometimes ask me if they were looking any different as labour approached (for instance, if their belly looked bigger or had shifted downwards slightly, which often happens as a baby engages). This was because I had seen them each week whereas the team midwives rotated consultations, meaning I saw some women more regularly than each team midwife. At new born four-day checks and six-week postnatal check-ups I was often (very pleasantly) tasked with holding babies while their mothers were physically checked.

Sitting in consultations three days a week for a year, and meeting with women outside the consulting rooms, gave me the opportunity to become deeply acquainted with the rhythms of midwifery. The consultation room of five of the midwives in the study (one single midwife used the team practice rooms) had white cotton curtains and light cream walls. The room had boards covered with pictures of babies the midwives had delivered and on the mantelpiece were thank-you cards from clients. Typically, midwives welcomed a client with a broad smile and a 'how are you?' Daily annoyances and work issues were talked about and the midwives wove these conversations into ones on the actual pregnancy. Women were asked how they felt and a discussion on ailments of pregnancy emerged along with a reassuring explanation from the midwife and a smile of sympathy. Physical checks often included a physical touch from midwives – a hand placed on a women's shoulder or on her belly. Checks were done between conversations; the only check no spoke at was during the blood pressure reading, where midwives concentrated on the various aspects that had to be recorded for an accurate reading. Listening to the heartbeat, many women commented on how reassuring it was to hear and the midwives smiled back, using both the Doppler (a hand-held device used to listen to a baby's heartbeat) and their own sense of what sounded normal (midwives sometimes looked at the window and did not talk for a few seconds before saying 'it sounds perfect!'), to assess that all was 'right'.

With the increasing medicalisation of birth, approaches to pregnancy have changed: how an unborn child is imagined and how bonding occurs through new reproductive technologies, especially amniocentesis and scans. Rayna Rapp (1999: 119) describes how the signs of the progress of pregnancy are produced quickly when tracked via ultrasound and other kinds of medical technology. With visual technology, 'abnormalities' and seeing a baby for the first time in utero contribute to when pregnancy is known and how it is known and how a growing baby is understood and known by expecting parents and medical professionals (Han 2013). Yet, according to Rapp (1999) there are also (slower) embodied signs of pregnancy – slower to be made known in the course of a pregnancy as well as, perhaps, slower to recognise – such as changing scents, sore breasts, crying and dizziness. Signs of the progress of pregnancy may not occur in all pregnant women and may be subtle and not necessarily recognised, making the awareness of the progress of pregnancy slower. The question of temporality is important with regard to midwife-assisted births.[8] Midwives in my study did not use ultrasound or perform amniocentesis. They relied on tools that detect foetal heartbeat, feeling a woman's body, visual clues, counselling and listening to a women's experiences during pregnancy in order to track and monitor gestation. If problems were detected or women wanted further testing, the midwives would refer them for amniocentesis, although all women using midwives in this study had a back-up obstetrician who would perform an amniocentesis should it be required. Many of the women with whom I worked had chosen a midwife-attended birth because they did not want 'unnecessary' scans and felt that engaging with their baby did not need to happen visually, often reporting feeling more of a connection with their baby with the midwives who used tactile, embodied means of checking on babies – their hands, listening with a Doppler, which was not considered a form of technology aligned with obstetric-led birth (Morgan 2009: 25).

I witnessed how women changed over the course of the pregnancy, how they steadily became more comfortable with their midwife/midwives and how they went from enjoying pregnancy to wishing their babies out (despite the midwives regularly telling the women to be patient). I was able to observe the format of consultations and the ways in which conversations were held while physical checks were completed, and knew the routine so well that if a midwife was running a little late getting to the practice, I was jokingly asked when she arrived, why, instead of talking with clients, I had not sent women to do their urine sample. In between consultations the midwives and I spoke about the impressions we had of the women and who was likely to go into labour soon. It was during these brief conversations between clients that I got an insight into how the midwives felt and responded to their work.

Evans' (2010) study on the independent midwives in the Cape Peninsula found that of 836 women using a midwife between 2003 and 2009, the majority (74.9 per cent) were white, 21 per cent were Coloured, 3.8 per cent were black and 0.2 per cent were Indian. She also found that the majority of women were aged between thirty and forty. These data are apposite five years later: ten of the women in my study were aged below thirty and only two were over forty years old. The midwife practices were all based in the Southern Suburbs of Cape Town so most clients lived in the City Bowl, Southern Suburbs and the 'deep south' Cape Peninsula region. A few women came from the Northern Suburbs – an area considered to be on the outskirts of Cape Town in terms of the position of the city centre and South Peninsula entailing a 40–60 minute drive to the midwives' rooms, and with a smaller concentration of wealth compared to the city centre and Southern Suburbs – but this was less common as the midwives did not do home births or home visits in areas that were that far away, meaning that the women had to birth in hospital and come to the practice if they lived outside the suburb parameters that the midwives serviced postnatally.

The sample of women in the study were largely university trained with thirteen of the nineteen women having attended university and of those six were medically trained. Women came to their birthing decisions with a high level of knowledge and the skill set required for engaged research. For middle-class women, good mothering was equated with intensive mothering (see Waltz 2014, Faircloth 2009 and Avishai 2007 for an account of the shifts in modes of mothering from the good enough mother to the good mother and its history). Good mothering was connected strongly with being well informed about pregnancy, birth, babies and parenting. Women researched in detail the physiological processes of pregnancy, birth, breastfeeding, hormones and anatomy and knew about these processes. They used highly technical language in tracing their pregnancies and asking questions: a discursive agility that I found surprising given that few of those whom the midwives called 'clients' were medically trained.

The women with whom I worked sought to be good mothers 'from the start': that is, from as soon as they were able. For them, good mothering was about more than reading expert knowledge, it required an ability to question critically and reflexively multiple sources of information as an informed consumer (Murphy 1999 in Faircloth 2009). As Strathern (1995: 347) points out though, cultural life is lived via circulations of knowledge and, particularly, what is made known. Desiring a 'natural' birth, women were aware of the associated sets of knowledge at stake (they felt they had to be knowledgeable) and presumed (and were expected to know) in eliciting that birth. During the antenatal classes and doula training I attended, for example, I frequently heard that women needed to understand the physiology of birth in order to birth.

Insider/Outsider

As much as birth was women's work, it was work I had not done at the time of my fieldwork. Speaking with women and midwives who used their own experiences frequently to explain and describe pregnancy, birth and the early weeks of parenthood, I could only imagine these experiences. During the doula course, as the youngest participant, I was the only one not to have birthed. It was difficult to talk about birth when I could only relay my mother's or her close friends' experiences of birth and stories women had told me in fieldwork. I had a strong sense of how difficult the first few weeks of motherhood could be, how intense birth is and how easy it could be to miss postnatal depression, but I had not actually felt labour pain or found myself postnatally depressed.

I was an insider to beliefs about birth: I had internalised the natural/technical model of birth as binary. It was easy to have conversations with women about why birth was 'natural' and how particular ways of living and being appeared 'natural'. Internalising this model demonstrates how the natural/technical model is situated in wider forms of life that extend beyond birth choice. These were not personal stakes for me though: I was not pregnant and contemplating how I would give birth and so I was able to attend to the models in particular ways, turning a critical eye on how versions of birth were differentiated.

I found myself both insider and outsider. I am female and middle-class and that gave me relatively easy access into conversations with women. Most women were only a few years older than me, a few were my age. Yet the focus of the study, care in pregnancy and birth, were not experiences of my own. Narayan (1993) asks: how native is a native anthropologist? I was in many ways a native anthropologist: I lived ten minutes from the midwives' practice and near most of the women I interviewed. Challenges existed in terms of what I saw and heard as these were often familiar and therefore easy to take for granted; turns of phrase, general musings and complaints of life. But I was also thoroughly unfamiliar: I do not know what it feels like to need to empty my bladder every ten minutes as a baby weighs down in my pelvis, or the feeling of being kicked from inside by a growing foetus, or the worry and concern that unfold in the limit experience of crafting life. But having not given birth was in many ways helpful to my study. When women described birth, I needed to ask multiple questions to try and understand what they meant. The pain of birth is in many ways unspeakable and so rich narratives and metaphors emerged in our conversations. The delicate balance of being part of a world that I was distanced from in significant ways came to bear on fieldwork and data production.

A Note on Intervention

Bridget, the midwife who attended Rachel's pregnancy and birth, frequently said 'you have to work to get the birth you want'. She meant that women needed to exercise, eat well and sit/kneel/stand in positions to help their baby into an optimal position for birth, and then continuously practise those forms of work throughout pregnancy. While it is presented as 'natural' and inevitable in much of the literature on birth, so-called 'natural' birth is, in the model Bridget and others use, something that must be achieved through careful preparation to lessen technocratic 'intervention'.

Intervention became a marker of how a labour could and would unfold. Each midwife was biomedically trained and worked within biomedical parameters of safety management. In the model used by Bridget and her fellow midwives and their clients, natural birth should not need to be worked towards: at some point a body goes into labour and a baby might or might not emerge healthy and well. Yet intervention in versions of birth categorised as 'natural' was indeed part of these births. Sets of parameters described the optimal situation for 'intervention-free' birth. The baby should be a singleton, cephalic (in a position so that the baby's head emerges before its body), preferably left occipital anterior (baby's back is facing away from the woman's and facing the left side of the woman's body), and delivered before forty-two weeks gestation. The baby should measure a certain size and women with diabetes with babies having estimated weights of more than 4kgs were closely monitored as fat distributed on the baby's shoulders was an important factor in determining safe delivery. There needed to be a certain amount of amniotic fluid and women's blood pressure needed to be within a specific range. Blood glucose levels needed to measure below 11.1 mmol in a random blood glucose reading. The existence of safety parameters established a norm: there were physiological limits to whether or not women could have their desired 'intervention-free' births. The horizons of risk and safety were established, setting up the probabilities of intervention (free) births. The distinction between intervention and intervention-free rests on a particular idea and myth of what intervention is (as I will show) and establishes the binary of natural and technocratic/medicalised birth that is the basis upon which women make birthing 'choices'.

The myth, and its binary, were powerful in producing the versions of care made available by midwives. It also drew attention to birth rather than the baby during pregnancy and women spent hours working on their birth plans, imagining and envisaging their desired birth. As 'technocratic' (or, as it was more commonly termed, 'biomedical' or 'medicalised') and 'natural' birth myths existed as one another's other, the midwives worked to produce a kind of care that they, along with their clients, believed to be largely unavailable in the obstetrician-led and medicalised birth sector, despite the fact that the midwives were positive about the kind of care given by some obstetricians, especially the four who backed them up.

The Way Forward

My study provides an account of a desired version of 'everyday', 'personalised' care in which care-receivers were not ill or in economically precarious situations, but were receiving care in a clinical setting and a formalised quality of antenatal care. I draw attention to what care can mean and look like in this setting.

In the context of elite health care, women were paying for a kind of care. Not only did they want care that facilitated and materialised a version of their desired birth, they also wanted care to look and feel a certain way. Everyday familiarity and relationality were key markers of desired care. Care happens in the everyday with particular limits, fluctuations and boundaries; this book pays attention to a specific, temporally limited care relationship of pregnant women and midwives, in which a version of care was modelled on everyday notions of 'familiarity' and 'personalised' care.

I look at how those relations are constituted. Generalised care that facilitated many births was simultaneously made specific as women called for flashes of midwives' personalities, hints of the everyday nuisances and joys of life, and companionability. I offer an account and an enrichment of the idea of care as an 'everyday problem' in a formalised setting of care work (Han 2012). In asking what makes care and a care-giver, I draw attention to how care-receivers were part of the crafting of the intimate life of care.

Noting Joel Robbin's (2013) suggestion that anthropology's focus on suffering in the forms of pain, poverty, violence and oppression, takes attention away from other aspects of daily life, and southern African anthropology has largely followed suit. In the aftermath of gross injustices, post-Apartheid cultural life is inflected with deep inequalities, violence, structural violence and for many people, is very hard work (Ross 2010). Southern African anthropologists have largely and necessarily turned their attention to engaging with the struggles and precarity of everyday life. My study came out of an interest in midwifery, and a concern about the reports of inadequate care in the public sector, as I have described above. There were plenty of reports and studies of inadequate and 'bad' care but this did not answer the question of what 'good', adequate or different versions of care might mean. By looking at a case study where women reported satisfaction with the care they received, I hoped to look at 'good' care and draw attention to a middle-class setting, an understudied aspect of anthropological enquiry; thus, my work offers an intervention into southern African anthropology and draws attention to questions of who anthropologists study and why. Southern African anthropology does not often turn attention to 'studying up' (Nader 1969), which is indeed the focus of this book. Francis Nyamnjoh (2015) critiques 'anthropology's object' – the pristine object of study in which questions of being an insider/outsider and how one studies one's 'own' is considered. The topic of study in this ethnography offers a move away from studying 'the poor' and draws attention to studying middle-class life and the questions of reflexivity and objects of study critical in contemporary anthropological debates.

Most importantly perhaps, my work offers an account of the spread of a global imaginary of positive birthing. The context of unique health systems and racial inflection in everyday life means that birthing in South Africa has its own nuanced concerns and challenges. Yet the travelling of birth models settles locally and informs women's daily birth desires and affects the ways in which birth is spoken of, imagined and practised. My book offers an account of the local settling of a global imaginary in a local context. As Kelly (2013) writes of Han's (2012) work on care in Chile and the ways in which people care for one another and their drug-using kin in the everyday, it is not that privilege, inequality, jealousy and cruelty, amongst other factors and emotions, do not exist in life, but that generosity and care exist alongside and part of these aspects of life. My study focuses on such qualities in the midst of deeply racialised, stratified care networks.

An overarching myth informed by historical, political and economic discourse comes to bear on how women imagined and constructed cultural storylines that produced a myth-making process of dichotomised versions of birth. These models hinge on various understandings and definitions of intervention. In Chapter 1 I describe the myth of birth that was informed and crafted by women desiring 'natural' birth and the ways that 'natural' and 'medicalised' birth are one another's other. The chapter offers an account of how this was indeed a myth and not a discourse, an elaboration of models of birth and how the models come to bear on the ways pregnancy and birth were imagined. Chapter 2 attends to the ways in which women engaged with pregnancy as plan. I describe how women approached knowledge, risk and choice in terms of a plan and I argue that the pregnancy as plan operates as a method for instantiating a kind of visibility as women did 'good' women's work. The chapter examines how women were able to plan how they would birth, tracing the privilege of choice and planning. Chapter 3 offers an account of the language used and the pain stories women told as they anticipated birth. Using Faye Ginsburg's (1987) model of procreation stories, I argue that the moral dimensions inflecting birthing choices were defined by experiencing and mediating painful childbirth. A racial stratification along lines of rural and urban birthing was connected with pain and self, and the chapter explores these dynamics. Thus, the chapter describes the ways in which an ethics of the self was constituted as women accounted for pain as 'character-developing' work. Classes, preparations and metaphor are, I argue, techniques of the self that were part of the ethics of the self at stake in life-giving work. Chapter 4 provides an insight into how birthing relations are made and how women who are white in South Africa are able to choose their care providers and the series of affects that inflect their care. The powerful moral underpinning of birth, and particularly 'natural' birth, reflects a construction of the self at stake. Care and birthing relations provided a means to self-care. In this chapter I look closely at how care relations such as trust, familiarity and intimacy are made in relation to the attentions and experiences women anticipated. I show how middle-class reproductive life is imagined as individual work rather than one shared in an extended social network. Thus, the chapter attends to the ways in which care offers intimacy in collective life, as a service. I show how the separations of the private and public sphere are offset in liberal democratic life. In the concluding chapter I draw together the themes of care, choice, privilege and race, to show how care and birthing practices are part of a broader network of privilege. Race and privilege remain closely connected in South Africa, and my study offers an ethnographic account of how race is reproduced in health care. To begin, I grapple with the myths of birth and the ways in which the boundaries of 'natural' and 'medicalised' birth are blurred.

Notes

1. Medical aid or medical insurance is a monthly payment plan offered by medical insurance companies in South Africa. One pays a monthly fee (which varies depending on what option is chosen in accordance with high or low medical needs), and when a medical procedure or medication is necessary, medical aid carries the cost. Some options require a shortfall payment as some hospitals and medical professionals practising in the private sector charge more than medical aid rates (determined each year), even up to 400% above these rates.
2. See study by Visagie and Posel (2011).
3. South Africa has a Gini coefficient of 0.63 according to the World Bank (2011), one of the highest in the world, with 1 being the measure of the greatest discrepancy.
4. In the book I use the term 'natural birth' to describe both how women defined a 'natural' birth (vaginal birth unmedicated) and the broad ideas informed by and informing the model of 'natural birth' as universally feminine, women's work. In Chapter 1, I elaborate on the model known as the 'natural birth' model.
5. The global call from health practitioners concerned about high C-section rates has, however, led to WHO affirming the need to review the 1985 statement on C-section rates.
6. This percentage is still above WHO's recommendations and may be linked to the older average age of clientele in my study as well as care

providers who take a more 'conservative' approach to birth due to high insurance costs.

7. All names have been changed in this study.
8. According to the webpage for the midwives at The Cape Town Midwives, 'consultations allow time for questions and are usually 30 minutes in duration. We always welcome partners to attend the consultations to stay as involved as possible throughout the pregnancy'.

Chapter 1

MYTHS OF BIRTH

INTERVENTION, HAVING 'CHOICE' AND HISTORIES OF BIRTH

The ways in which women access, and, critically, their ability to access versions of care in South Africa, have a strong historical component and are shaped by a colonial and Apartheid legacy. The racialised stratifications of medical care in South Africa at present are entrenched in the devastating effects of racial segregation. I explore this history here. I also grapple with the myths of birth that are closely aligned to a historical and racially-based romanticisation of birthing 'naturally'. In this chapter, I trace how a bifurcated model of birth emerged, where 'natural' and 'medicalised' birth were established as starkly different from one another. Yet, I will show how the two are one another's other. I will also show how the myth of dichotomised birth models is shaped and inflected by South Africa's racialised history, how this plays out at present in the form of private and public health sectors, and who is able to access certain kinds of care.

The ways women in my study approached birth were not orientated around safety and survival, an unusual fact in a country with high maternal and infant mortality rates. Rather, birth was approached as a choice-based practice. In this context privilege is about choice; it is also about ignorance.

'Choosing' How to Birth

For the small group of women who chose an independent midwife as their primary care provider during pregnancy, the desired outcome was to birth 'naturally'. Women seeking a 'natural' birth understood their bodies to be designed to birth in a particular way, and understood it to be a 'natural' process that had occurred for millennia. Women wanted a 'natural' birth and they spoke about safety concerns, but conversations on birth often failed to factor in that the means by which safe outcomes were ensured was the availability of medicalised back-up, deemed 'unnatural', should a birth go awry. Women using midwives saw themselves as fighting against the capitalistic, medicalised, technocratic and surgical style of birth in South Africa's private sector and against what they perceived as the generalised perception from the medicalised community that 'natural' birth was dangerous and midwives were not the safest option as birth attendants. Women in my study saw birth as a 'natural' event and therefore an inevitable one. Absent from their birthing talk was the fact that these women were able to choose how they birthed. This choice reflects enormous privilege.

The South African private health sector provides women who have medical aid with the 'option' of how they birth; most women using private health care have their pregnancy attended to by an obstetrician, a specialist surgeon in pregnancy, who engages with birth and its complications. The obstetrician, as a medical professional, is able to facilitate surgical birth in the form of C-sections, the births 'in between' (forceps and ventouse) and vaginal birth. High C-section numbers suggest that the choice to have an elective C-section was a popular one. Yet having the perception of choice was not as simple as it appeared. Fact merged with fiction and varying imaginings crafted a perception of a divided birthing private sector.

Tess Cosslett (1994) is critical of the medicalised/natural birth binary. She demonstrates the ways in which medicalised and 'natural' birth discourses are both anti-feminist and rely on a myth of primitive, essential motherhood – a non-specific universal (black) woman born to birth. That there are two competing birth stories is, for Cosslett, potentially a cultural myth. Scholarship on birth seeks to differentiate the two (see Rich 1976, Davis-Floyd 1992, Jordan 1978, Martin 1987, Kitzinger 1992, 2002, 2005, Chadwick and Foster 2013, Chadwick et al. 2014).

In this chapter, I take an alternate route, describing how women spoke about these models. The literature on birth has tended to set up stark contrasts between 'medicalised' and 'natural' birth, the former framed as a domain where women's bodies are controlled by male doctors and the latter existing as a sphere belonging, metaphorically, to women alone. A mode of restoration underpins the natural birth model, an event aligned with nature but, since the advent of modern medicine, one that has been appropriated by technology and medicalised ideas of birthing. Instead, I am interested in how conversations overlapped and imaginings of stark differences were contradicted by actual experience. Cosslett (1994) argues that the models of birth are a discourse as they have had the power to shape the way in which childbirth is practiced. As I will show though, how childbirth unfolded, where and with whom did not fall within the neat boundaries of two models of birth. Rather, the boundaries were blurred. The chapter therefore offers an account of the two models of birth as one another's other. I explore the idea of intervention as a marker of different versions of birth. In rethinking 'intervention' and what intervention means, the ideas constituting 'natural' and medical births become less obviously distinguished, offering an ethnographic account of women's experiences in relation to academic birthing narratives.

Claude Levi-Strauss' (1978) idea of the stitching together of pieces of myths and mythemes, each with their own histories that come to inform and tell a story, is a useful one, despite its critiques. The stitching of patchwork pieces of narrative offers an avenue into thinking about relations and connections that come together to produce cultural storylines that shape birthing and care (Strathern 1988). I show how birthing myths appeared as a binary, but I also show that the binaries were contradicted, blurred and modulated by various aspects of social life. I describe the various renderings of birth talk and beliefs, and how the connections between these come to animate women's birthing ideals (Strathern 1988).

The ways histories and myth come to shape and produce choice is critical here. The conflation of history and myth shows how a powerful myth-making process upheld a binary of medicalised versus natural birth. 'Choice' became the axis on which women approached birth, established via a binary of birth models. There were multiple storylines and histories, imagined and real, that produced ideas of birth and of which kinds of people birthed in particular ways. Coupled with this, the modernist separation of nature and culture produced a specific rendering of 'the natural' and what it meant to birth naturally outside the realms of medical intervention. Ideas of safety, risk and consumer-driven capital imperatives all came to act upon beliefs around birth. The chapter thus teases out the overlaps and connectedness of the myth-making processes that produced birthing ideals via the myth being hinged on notions of intervention, scientific discourse and biomedical training. Therefore, while I show that a birth myth existed, I am interested in the relations, connections, disconnections and contradictions in birth talk for those able to 'choose' how to give birth.

A South African History of Birth and Its Medicalisation

In order to grapple with the myth presently, it is necessary to look at the history of birth in South Africa, which comes to inform the way birth talk is constituted by a myth and spoken of in terms of choice. Middle-class women using independent midwives 'chose' to birth without what they understood as medical intervention. Not having to engage with the challenges faced by those in the public health sector, middle-class women focused their attention on the challenges of birthing for those in private care: a scenario in which close to seventy per cent of women have C-sections (SAHR 2013: 241). As such, women using independent midwives came to conversations on birth with particular framings and politics around birth. They saw themselves fighting against the perceived notion that C-sections were a largely inevitable outcome of giving birth in the private sector. Their ideas about how they wanted to birth soon took centre stage in their imaginings of the pregnancy.

In the colonial history of South Africa, nursing developed unofficially with Dutch women taking care of the ill in communities and family members nursing each other (Digby and Sweet 2005). In 1687, Aletta Kaisers became the first midwife on record: the Dutch East India Company, which established Cape Town as a rest stop, needed licensed midwives but as people began to relocate beyond the confines of the city, the Company midwife could not attend to the needs of all women. There were so few midwives in the 1700s that if one died, another had to be sent out from Europe. To obviate this need, Dutch settler women and men were eventually trained. By 1825 there were twenty-three accoucheurs (male birth attendants who were usually medical doctors) and sixteen midwives in the Colony (there had been only one in 1807 [Searle 1965: 99]). There were, however, still many women practising as midwives without formal training. The licensing of midwives began under

Dutch control – women were sent out from the Netherlands – although local midwives remained unlicensed. Rather than using local women, unlicensed but not necessarily unknowledgeable, midwives were sent to the Colony. Instead, local women (particularly black women) were represented as 'dirty' and 'incapable' because they lacked formal training, and racial and gender divides were established along the lines of skilled/trained vs. unskilled/untrained practitioners. It was only in the late nineteenth century in the Cape Colony, now under British control, that white British nurses came to South Africa. Religious sisterhoods were involved in nursing and the notion of nursing as a respectable profession began to develop when nurses' training was established in Kimberley in the late 1870s. These practices could vary across regions however, given that South Africa had Dutch and British controlled areas, but there were also Boer republics and other political groupings, where medical care would have not been regulated in the same ways.

Harriet Deacon (1998) explores the power relations between men and women in the Cape Colony in the early 1800s, showing how birth became medicalised. Male accoucheurs were marketed as the choice for upper-class women in Europe and Britain in the 1700s. There, the introduction of the forceps improved the reputations of accoucheurs, as under their ministrations there were more live births than was the case with midwives who did not use forceps. The influence of positive birth rates via forceps was felt in the Cape, where accoucheurs also began to be used. The training of midwives and certification by Cape doctors helped to regulate the practice, positioning women as junior partners rather than competitors (Deacon 1998: 274). This was because doctors, in training midwives, could be seen to possess superior knowledge and the former pattern of apprenticeship of new midwives to old midwives began to dissipate.

In 1810, Johann Wehr, a doctor, started a midwifery school at the Slave Lodge in Cape Town (Searle 1965). Despite an attempt to make use only of licensed midwives, the 1840s 'still' saw 'Malay girls' attending births as unofficial birth attendants. Wehr's son was dismayed at this as he felt it was dangerous, and began training midwives. By 1849, he had trained thirteen more (Deacon 1998: 278). The emphasis was not on education and empowerment but on regulation and creating a 'respectable' group of women, divided along racial lines. So while midwives were made subservient to medical doctors, they were still seen as legitimate members of 'respectable' society. Here, the emergence of a connection between respectability and official licensing was established. The way in which care is practised is also foregrounded: 'unofficial' birth attendants were framed as unknowledgeable and lacking in biomedical training, whereas licensed carers were figured as respectable, safe members of the medical community. It is necessary to note that this is a history of white, colonial society – how women were cared for during childbirth in other sectors is largely unrecorded but would likely have existed as apprenticeship style training. Thus, notions of 'official' training, respectability and race became aligned.

Racialised differentiation was increasing by the 1830s. While white midwives were acceptable to (white) English women living in the city, black women were almost non-existent in annual published medical almanacs and directories, as middle- to upper-class women either consulted white English midwives or accoucheurs. Doctors, seeking more work, also entered into the field of birthing (Deacon 1998: 286). British immigrants preferred accoucheurs while Dutch immigrants tended to work more with black women and adopted the birthing practices of Khoi San women, for instance, using teas and herbs to help facilitate and initiate labour and birth. In this way, ethnic and racial cleavages began to emerge. Class divides too began to be established, running especially along racial lines. Competition between doctors and midwives was limited (most doctors practised in the city) largely because (male) doctors remained in upper-class areas while midwives operated in poorer areas. Strong class, race and gender differentiations in the distribution of services began to be consolidated. An initial concern about black midwives (as poorly trained and incompetent) took the focus away from (white) licensed midwives who were, by extension, able to continue their work.

By the end of the nineteenth century however, attention had turned to poor (Afrikaans) white midwives too (Deacon 1998: 292, Digby and Sweet 2005). In 1894, over 200 women applied to train at Kimberley's midwifery school, marking a clear professionalisation of birthing practices (Searle 1965: 28). Whereas health care had previously been conducted primarily in the home, with care given by relations, friends and servants, the British colonial government of the mid-nineteenth century decided that this was high-risk and placed too much of a burden on families, legislating the need for licensing. As nursing was moved from the home to hospital, women (but only a certain kind) were required. Birth, conflated with primal qualities – a 'monstrous' event (see Cosslett 1994), part of 'women's' domain, uncontrollable and the territory of apprenticed but unofficially trained women – established associations with midwifery. Licensed, trained midwives became associated with respectable work that moved birth from being a messy, dangerous event, to one that could be sanitised, in hospital and dealt with by trained carers. A rhetoric of the 'good woman' had become prevalent by the mid-nineteenth century. A 'good' woman took no pay and did the work out of willingness alone, as a gentlewoman. 'Disciplined', 'self-sacrificing', 'moral' and 'ethical' were the terms applied to nursing, which attracted many women as it was a 'respectable' paid profession. This was amplified by the fact that religious sisterhoods were the first nurses; a conflation of nursing and femininity began to occur, which was later attached to the self-sacrificing rhetoric of women in health care. The conflation created both gender divisions and a sense of the self-sacrificing woman, constructing a model of obligation in which women needed to be good and giving, and work for no money, while continuing to care for others: the mothering model was moved into the public sector and formal care. As Marks (1994) and Packard (1996) show, race, gender and class intersected in the twentieth century as black women and white Afrikaans women fought for respect in the male-dominated profession of medicine during Apartheid. At the same time, these women were working toward upward class mobility. A racialised, class-based political economy of birthing, framed in terms of care and biomedical knowledge, was consolidated.

These themes have informed the debates around birth in multiple contexts. Conversations began to emerge around safety and the use of technology. Doctors began using forceps for the first time in the nineteenth century and the mid-twentieth-century medicalisation emphasised medicine and science as the salvation from the dangers of birth. Indeed, salvation was necessary with the infant mortality rate at 196 per 1000 births between 1837 and 1909 in South Africa (Katzenellenbogen and Dorrington 1993). Sanitised (using technology and analgesia), medicalised birth became part of a narrative in which birth was understood as a dangerous event to be mediated by medicalised processes undertaken by doctors to ensure safety (Chadwick 2007). Shaped by racialised, gendered and class separation of Afrikaaner and black women birthing rurally under the care of a non-medically trained person and white, upper-class English women who were able to access the safety, control and cleanliness of hospital birth. The issue of how one birthed and who cared for labouring women took on importance. Historically speaking, as birth care moved in the twentieth century from women carers and the home to hospitals, a powerful rhetoric of hospitals being safer because doctors and surgical intervention were available should problems arise emerged and has been maintained in perceptions of birth in South Africa (Lapperman 2011). Thus, South Africa's present birthing practices reflect historical imperatives that have constructed birth as a medicalised event.

Birthing continues to operate on the racial and class lines upon which health care is accessed in South Africa, reinforced by perceptions of the natural and ideas of the 'rural' in natural births. The romanticised understanding of rural woman birthing with ease in the fields, along with the rhetoric of 'natural' birth, produces a fetishised image and body of the natural. Mcleod and Durrheim (2002) provide a historical overview of how biological 'scientific' racism was replaced in Apartheid-era South Africa with notions of 'culture', 'tradition' and 'ethnicity' and how these terms began to perform the work of 'race' categories. Indeed, these categories – running in parallel with the segregation of people in provinces and Bantustans – made health care a service that, for non-white South Africans, was not only differentiated according to race and class, but also according to where one lived and the Bantustan one was categorised as being part of. Ethnicity and tradition, amplified by the use of Bantustans, were made to do kinds of work in terms of instantiating racial 'stereotypes'. McLeod and Durrheim (2002) write that in terms of pregnancy this was

> achieved in the South African literature on teenage pregnancy through (1) the portrayal of 'blacks' as possessing 'culture' with 'whites' having what Wetherell and Potter (1992: 71) call a 'mundane, technical and practical outlook' and (2) the construction of a dichotomy between the 'traditional' and the 'modern' with the 'traditional' implicitly meaning 'black' and the 'modern' implying 'white'. (Mcleod and Durrheim 2002: 12)

Fassin and Schneider (2003), in an analysis of HIV/AIDS perceptions, provide similar findings. They show how racialisation (and in South Africa, geographical separation) is rooted in history, with health used as a means to separate people along race lines. With a distinct history of racialised bodies, the image of the rural, black women birthing naturally became a symbolic means for those desiring a 'natural birth' of thinking through the 'naturalness' of birth. For women who opted for elective C-sections, the rural as a symbol of 'natural' was again framed in the negative, as unruly and primitive (Lapperman 2011); the hospital became a safe, sanitised space where order and control were maintained. The women in my study who wanted a particular version of vaginal birth drew on a storyline in which 'the natural', conflated with the notion of rural birthing and primality, was used as a narrative for why birth should be 'natural'.

As the medicalisation of birth increased, international debates about models of birth emerged. The popular literature on birthing in South Africa is not extensive, but the international literature has played a role in how birth materialises and is imagined by middle-class South African women using midwives presently.

International Debates on Birth: Feminism, Rights, Technologised Birth

While conflicting views on birth have existed for centuries, the interest in birth models, specifically technocratic/medicalised models, became popular in the 1960s and 1970s with the surge in feminist movements in the United States and the United Kingdom (Oakley 1979, Katz Rothman 1982, MacCormack 1982, Kitzinger 1962). Specifically, birth emerged as an anthropological topic of inquiry in its own right, rather than simply appearing as part of the life-cycle, when Brigitte Jordan published *Birth in Four Cultures* in 1978, a cross-cultural analysis of the ways in which birth is viewed in the United States, the Netherlands, Sweden and Yucatan. Jordan demonstrated that birth is not only a physiological event; birth is understood and approached as a cultural practice. Jordan offered an account of birth that foregrounded the dismantling of singular understandings of birth and called for scholarship that focused on birthing practice as a specific site of enquiry. Her intervention inaugurated a productive period. Written largely by women, the birth literature of the 1960s and 1970s focused mainly on the patriarchal framing of birth, critiquing the powerful rhetoric that so-called 'medicalised birth' produced safer births and better outcomes. The literature presented the problems with medicalised birth procedures, such as women feeling disempowered during labour, and what many writers saw as unnecessary medical and surgical interventions in the form of unrequested analgesia, episiotomy, ventouse and forceps delivery, and C-sections. In the United States, where much of this literature emerged, midwifery and feminism became aligned.

However, not all researchers polarised medical versus 'natural' birth models. Oakley (1980) and Kitzinger (1962) understood 'natural' birth to be an event that was thought and spoken about in medicalised terms. They argued that birth was not 'natural' because it was not women-centred in the sense that labouring women were supposedly left out of decision-making processes and were subjected to 'unnecessary intervention'. Thus, their arguments suggest that the category 'natural' should not bc understood solely in terms of physiology but in terms of the social formations of care and attention; a truly natural birth is not just a vaginal delivery but a process centred on women's agency. Yet they still understood 'natural' birth as a distinct category. Feminist (natural) birth writers understood birth to be a natural process for women to experience alongside other women, without the control of (male) doctors, although definitions of 'natural' birth remained vague. Certain feminist authors and midwives argued that birth needed to be moved back into the realm of women-centred and women-supported births and in so doing established a (perhaps inadvertent) dichotomy between medical and 'natural' birth (see Kitzinger 1962 and Katz Rothman 1982).

Katz Rothman (1982) and Ginsburg and Rapp's (1995) critiques of medicalised birth (understood at this time as hospital births where women were confined to bed and given analgesia and synthetic oxytocin as standard practice) centred on women's bodies framed not only as aberrations from the male norm (pregnancy, birth and lactation therefore became pathological), but also in technological terms – birthing as a problem that was technical and required technical solutions. Technology and medicine became conflated in the birthing literature, with 'technocratic' and 'medicalised' births used as interchangeable terms. Because birth preparation classes, an emergent intervention (i.e. classes have not always existed but are presumed as a norm for many women presently) at the time (1960s), were highly formalised, they were also categorised as part of the medicalised model of birth.

For these feminist birth writers of the United States and Britain, natural birth on the other hand was seen to be midwife-led, and pregnancy was not understood as an illness but as a life stage. They argued that the birthing process did not require preparation because it was innate to women's bodies (Katz Rothman 1982). Cosslett (1994: 15) shows how male proponents of 'natural' birth such as Grantly Dick-Read (1933) (see below) saw 'natural' birth as an event to be controlled by the mind. Part of his argument was that pain was 'unnatural' and therefore if women experienced pain they were doing something 'wrong'. For Dick-Read, the mind had been overly 'civilised' by contemporary living and this prevented the 'primal' part of women from labouring 'as nature intended'. Cosslett argues that that control was seen to be in the hands of (male) doctors; she goes on to suggest that a further appropriation happened as women attempted to 'control' birth in different ways. Female scholars' appropriation of natural birth, by Kitzinger (1962), attempted to move the doctors' 'control of the mind' to labouring women. Cosslett (1994: 20) argues that both arguments relied on the myth of 'the primitive woman' and 'male medicine', setting up a contrast between two models of birth. Cosslett shows how each model deployed elements of the other, for example induction in some cases was regarded as 'natural'.

Cosslett uses 'the primitive woman' to explain how the ideas of 'natural' birth and medicalised birth are part of the same myth: both rely on a specific understanding of women, either needing to be saved from primitive birth or restored. I attempt to expand on this point by showing how the myths of birth are imbricated in the work and care of midwives and in acknowledging the midwife as a form of intervention.

Moving to the birth literature of the 1990s, Robbie Davis-Floyd (1992) argues that birth has moved from being a women-focused experience to a model founded on an 'ideology of technological progress', and that technocratic birth movements and their associated rites and rituals take away women's power over their bodies, which are 'naturally' designed to birth. Birth, according to Davis-Floyd, presents a 'conceptual threat to male dominance'. She suggests that medical rituals (such as placing women in wheelchairs as they arrive at hospital, symbolically telling women they are disabled) have been created to make medical staff feel like they are the producers of the babies rather than the women. She argues that society has designed obstetric rituals to deliver nature (vaginal birth) into culture (via intervention and C-section births). She goes on to suggest that to empower women, 'choice' should be at the forefront of birthing. For Davis-Floyd, the body-mind dualism is maintained in medicalised births and these distinctions rest on a conceptual separation of nature and culture. Yet those scholarly separations inform and become part of the myth of birth, reinforcing ideas of birthing models as opposed. An attempt to move away from the reinforcing ideas of birth included emphasising the voice of women in feminist birth literature (Klassen 2001). Lou-Marie

Kruger (2003), writing on South African women's experiences of motherhood, suggests that even when individual stories are used to subvert myths of birth and motherhood, she found that women internalised and replicated dominant ideologies. As such, Kruger argues that individual stories are shaped by political ideologies and ambivalence cannot be expressed because it does not form part of the main birthing and motherhood narratives. Likewise, Chadwick and Foster (2013) show how women's risk constructions were related to three specific birthing embodiments: technocratic bodies, vulnerable bodies and knowing bodies. Each group at different times endorsed and subverted the biomedical model of birth and risk. While Chadwick (2007, Chadwick et al. 2014) argues that embodied knowledge to some degree subverts medical models of birth, what is not emphasised is that embodied knowing can be framed within the 'natural' model of birth. Indeed, Chadwick's (2018) recent book argues that birth literature needs to focus more attention on 'the fleshy, embodied' aspects of birth. Yet, as I will show, an embodied way of knowing can be understood as part of a narrative in which natural birthing knowledge and 'intuition' inform a broader set of capitalist orientations to life and care. As such, it is clear that contemporary, local literature on birth still grapples with the powerful binary of birth models. The history of birthing and its associated medicalisation alongside the debates on birthing models come to inform present understandings and availabilities of birth for many middle-class women and indeed the medical system in South Africa.

'It Shouldn't Be Unnatural to Have Natural Birth': Views on Birth

Sasha had booked an appointment to see the Cape Town Midwives now that she was pregnant with her second child. She had used an obstetrician for her first birth and had been deeply dissatisfied by the birth because it had not unfolded as she had hoped and she felt out of control. During the consultation she was emotional: she cried as she talked about her first birthing experience and gestured anxiously, waving her hands frequently, speaking quickly, her face flushed. Beth, the midwife, listened to Sasha speak, offering her tissues as she cried. Sasha said: 'I was never given the chance to have natural, I want to try, but doctors get a sick pleasure out of cutting women open'.

Her strong language was striking. Assigning a sadomasochistic quality to doctors, Sasha's comment, while extreme, is indicative of how many women with whom I worked saw 'technocratic' birth in South Africa.

Gill, for example, had come to Bridget after having had a C-section that she believed was unnecessary. She described her first birth as traumatising because she felt 'out of control' and was given little power in the decision-making process as her birth plans unravelled. I visited Gill in her home when her baby was six weeks old. Gill sat on the floor with her daughter in front of her on a blanket describing her experiences. She said:

> I speak to people now and tell them I had natural birth and they're like wow, without any drugs? And I say yes and they say oh my word, you are amazing – like they'd almost treat me like a freak because it's something you don't hear and I think it's so sad – it's so sad, I almost want to cry cos all these people come to me and say I couldn't have a natural so I'm booking myself in for a caesarean section. I feel so strongly about it – I want to tell everyone who is pregnant, go with a midwife! It's really opened my mind to see what's going on in our country and how wrong it is. And it shouldn't be unnatural to have natural birth.

Women like Sasha and Gill were contrasting an imagining of natural birth against all the interventions and procedures they saw as overly medicalised and unnecessary. Gill and Sasha's views on medicalised birth imply it was the 'wrong' way to birth and suggest a moralistic mode of differentiation, illustrated in Sasha's comment that doctors got 'pleasure' from cutting women. Women like Gill and Sasha also described C-sections as the 'easy-route' to having a baby. What they negated in their understanding was that a C-section is abdominal surgery and the procedure and recovery time is harder in many ways. The work of their midwives became largely invisible in their imaginings and experiences of 'natural' birth via a powerful contrast of birth options.

It is important to note that for all women using private health care, a consumer-driven model of birthing was at stake and choice was rendered as a question of satisfaction. Women believed they were choosing their birth and were paying for that birth; they were therefore entitled to be satisfied with that birth. When they were not happy with an outcome, 'choice' and being 'out of control' became the language set used. This demonstrates the consumer-driven approach to birth in the private sector (Taylor 2000,

Hanson 2004). Paying for care was part of the consumer-driven behaviour of the women in my study and each woman using a midwife signed an indemnity form showing that they understood the risks and responsibilities of using midwife-led care (although the Consumer Protection Act did not affect the midwives). Yet despite signing these indemnity forms, women still saw the care they received as a right.[1]

Biomedicine as a form of authoritative knowledge has been well documented (Davis-Floyd and Sargent 1997, Farquhar 2012, Lambert 1992). Medical anthropologists and science studies scholars have closely interrogated the ways in which science works to legitimise certain ways of knowing over others, and which forms of knowledge count (Strathern 1995). As the nature/culture divide that began to separate knowledges became more powerful in the twentieth century, technology was aligned with culture and medicalised birth: it was considered safer because it controlled the uncontrollable (women, birth and nature) and was seen as being objective. Understandings of women being more closely aligned to nature and men to culture (Ortner 1972) underpinned and fuelled the ideas about the unruliness of women and birth, which was envisaged as being able to be safely controlled by medicalised, sanitised hospital birth. The perception of the controlled medicalised birth became more widely held.

Anthropological critiques of biomedicine are well established. Lock and Nguyen (2010) examine the dominance of biomedicine, noting its assumption that all bodies are the same and that disease is expressed, understood and experienced similarly. They also point to the extensive work on how biomedical technologies have been transferred to various settings, and how biomedical technology plays out differently at local sites. Bodies have been shown to stretch, move and meld in varying ways, meaning that cultural apparatuses act upon bodies and how people live in the world; Farmer (1996), Lock (1993), Scheper-Hughes (1987) all show the ways in which bodies are produced by and in the social. Thus, there are two models of the body presented in birthing literature and perceptions: the 'natural' and the 'biomedical'. Both imagine a (different) universal body: one, a woman's body unconstrained by culture, the other, an anatomically standard body. Lock and Nguyen (2010) present an intervention that allows the distinctions between a 'natural' and 'biomedical' body to be blurred. Women in my study actively modulated their birthing choices and ideas across these differentiating lines.

The work of undoing the hegemony of biomedicine has been necessary in allowing for alternate ways of knowing, different ways bodies are crafted and practice life and are acknowledged, allowing for the questioning of the meanings of 'truth' and objectivity. Yet, the assumption of biomedicine as a single, socially constructed, monolithic entity has also been critiqued. Good and Good (1993), drawing on Mulkay and Gilbert (1982), suggest that science studies often do not recognise the nuances and the multiple ways and versions in which the sciences operate. When biomedicine is lumped in with 'science' in general, critiques levelled at it can be guilty of forgoing the different ways in which doctors work, and their individual motivations and feelings within the institutional parameters of their work. Thus, Good and Good (1993) provide an insight into the ways in which biomedicine and its practitioners were set up as a generalised group offering standard versions of birth. Yet, women engaged the services of biomedically trained midwives who focused on their clients in nuanced and varying ways.

Women with whom I worked positioned obstetricians as surgeons eager to perform unnecessary C-sections but as Good and Good (1993) note, the individual feelings of doctors were rarely factored into women's accounts of doctors. However, each woman in my study had a back-up obstetrician who supported the midwives and supported women 'choosing' 'natural' birth. Good and Good (1993) shed some light on thinking about the complexity of these birth narratives: medicalised, technocratic birth models conflated doctors, institutions and understandings of medicalised birth. It is essential to note Good and Good's (1993) critique of the critiques of biomedicine and to acknowledge the subtleties that come to bear on birthing care. Indeed, doctors did not necessarily agree with the hospitals in which they worked not allowing midwives to work there too. Some obstetricians supported 'natural' birth but worked in a practice where the other doctors did not. The model of technocratic birth and those considered to be supporters of that model is more nuanced than it was made to seem in the accounts of pregnant women and in broader societal discourses. Over the course of my fieldwork, the obstetricians who backed up the midwives made the decision to no longer support VBAC (vaginal birth after C-section) midwife-assisted births. The midwives and women stated that this was a decision made by the obstetricians; this was true but it did not take into account other players and factors – the hospital and its managers, and potential pressure from insurance companies. Decisions were considered consolidated (as simple and final) by midwives; without acknowledging the layers and actors in choice-making for doctors, which were seen as one-dimensional even though this did not necessarily reflect the experiences and multiple relations of knowing that went into making that decision. There were specific parameters in place that determined whether women would 'get to birth as they desired'.

The divide in South Africa's private birthing sector is in many ways influenced by the debates that took 'natural' birth as a given. In the current South African context, midwives encourage and offer a particular kind of birth: 'normal', 'vaginal', VBACs and ideally without analgesia, C-sections or ventouse deliveries. A key term in the language around midwife-assisted birth was 'normal'. Midwives spoke of ligament pains being normal, a healthy sign of pregnancy, and reassured clients that feeling tired and getting stiff fingers towards the end of pregnancy was all part of the process, not to be worried about. Beth and Bridget both frequently said 'pregnancy is not an illness', Beth adding that she loved 'seeing women in a state of grace during pregnancy'. Part of the work of midwifery, according to the midwives, was 'to normalise pregnancy and the birth process'. Therefore, reassuring women and telling them their ailments were normal was an ordinary and essential part of consultations. Apart from the support of their midwife and partner, a normal birth was presented as entailing no medical intervention either surgically or in the form of analgesia, although birthing at home and at hospital were both counted as normal, even if most of the midwives preferred home births.

I have outlined the general framing from which a discourse of 'natural' versus medicalised birth emerged and how midwives approached birth from an understanding of it as 'normal'. The literature cited above, as well as clients and their midwives, differentiated medicalised birth from 'natural' birth along lines of intervention, on the basis that 'natural birth' did not require or involve intervention. Medical experiences were regarded as interventions to be avoided and midwife-assisted birth was seen by women as the best way to prevent intervention, by giving women time to labour, supporting them, encouraging doula support, and providing low lighting and a quiet space. Yet midwives themselves, and their varying practices, were not seen as interventions but as an extension of 'the natural', even when births occurred in hospital settings.

Midwives consistently encouraged clients to look at Spinning Babies (a website that detailed the positions women could get into to encourage optimal positioning of the baby and the woman's pelvic alignment for birth), showed them forward-leaning positions in consultations, to get the baby to be in an anterior rather than posterior position, walking to help positioning and labour, as well as a healthy diet for keeping blood pressure and blood glucose in check so that women would not develop the associated conditions that might prevent a vaginal delivery. Women needed to engage with these practices in order to get the births they wanted, something midwives reminded them of frequently.

There were strict parameters however, that guided when and if the versions of desired births would be possible. As biomedically trained medical professionals, midwives insisted that to birth vaginally under their care, certain conditions had to be met: that women were only carrying one baby; that the baby was not breech, that there was enough amniotic fluid, something that could be felt by midwives but was confirmed by a scan conducted by the required back-up obstetrician; that they delivered before forty-two weeks gestation; and that there were no jeopardising conditions such as pre-eclampsia and gestational diabetes. This was why women coming toward the end of their pregnancy were anxious if they had had a high blood pressure reading, some glucose in their urine, a measurement via ultrasound with their obstetrician (back-up obstetricians insisted their patients attend a thirty-seven-week consultation with them, as was part of the midwife-led care package) that indicated an 'abnormally' large baby (extra weight on the shoulders that can hinder delivery), or a baby that still had not turned from breech to cephalic (head down) at thirty-seven weeks.

Lily, for instance, was so concerned about her high blood pressure reading at her thirty-seven-week obstetric consultation that she bought a blood pressure monitor so she could check her blood pressure every few hours, anxious to see no signs of pre-eclampsia developing. Certain parameters allowed a certain kind of delivery and place of delivery (home or hospital). If those parameters did not exist, there would be no need to engage with issues of a breech baby, and no 'work' would be necessary in having a 'natural birth' outcome: labour would eventually begin and a baby would arrive well, or not. Women's anxiety towards the end of pregnancy demonstrated the limits around who could birth as they desired, 'naturally'.

Among midwives with whom I worked, women hoping for midwife-assisted births made use of both midwives and a back-up obstetrician: midwives were unwilling to support women without a back-up doctor. The distinction between models of 'natural' and 'technocratic' was blurred when a back-up obstetrician was used for a 'natural' birth. The above mentioned literature set obstetricians up as those who make birth technocratic and midwives as carers who enable 'natural' birth.[2] However, the safety net of a back-up physician is what allowed a 'natural' birth as a construct to exist as well as being a necessity if one used a registered independent midwife. The midwives in my study operated from a private hospital when women needed to be in hospital or did not want a home birth. In order to do so, they required back-up obstetric care and the obstetricians with whom they worked insisted on particular parameters of safety and required a consultation with their patient at the beginning and end of the pregnancy even if all was well. The intervention of the midwife (as an emergency trained professional and provider of particular kinds of care) was seen as 'natural' or not as intervention at all. Yet the midwives and obstetricians worked together, the latter supporting the former, and this destabilises the stark separation of natural/technical models of birth that I elaborate on below. Here, it becomes necessary to unpack carefully the myth of natural birth, the myth of biomedical birth and the myth of biomedical versus natural understandings of birth. The two models of birth would not exist without the other's myth; they have come to be one another's other.

Birthing Myths: The Myth of Biomedical Models of Birth

Emerging from modernist divisions of nature and culture, biomedicine has been crafted as the health practice of science, an authoritative knowledge assumed to be true, based in science and 'evidence' (Jordan 1978). Medical anthropologists and science studies scholars have written on how technology became conflated with culture and biomedicine, producing a narrative in which nature became steadily understood as separate from technology, and technologised birth and medicine were understood as better, more reliable and safer (Scheper-Hughes 1987, Lock 1993, Latour 2007). The body, particularly the female body, the original tool (Mauss 1935), became equated with nature.

When I asked midwives and pregnant women why they believed midwife-led birth to be the optimal choice, they spoke of how medicalised birth often meant labouring on one's back, in discomfort, being hooked up to a cardiotocography (CTG) machine. It also meant listening to the constant sound of machines and beeps, having bright lights and no privacy as unknown medical staff walked in to the labour room to check on the labour or bring drinks. Midwives recounted stories of how it was better to wait at home for as long as possible because labour would take a while but also, because once at hospital, in a stressful environment, labours had been known to slow down or stall. Women anticipated that when the obstetrician arrived for the delivery, they would be rushed to birth, and would likely experience intervention in the form of episiotomy or ventouse. Women felt that there would be little support should they have a medicalised birth as the hospital midwives worked on shifts and only checked labour progress; there would be little emotional support from them, nor from the doctors. Eighteen women spoke during consultations about their traumatic births, and said they had been uncared for, were left under bright lights and had little privacy. The atmosphere of medicalised birth was imagined and perceived as 'cold', 'clinical', 'public' and 'highly technologised'.

A generalised picture of a technocratic, medicalised birth was one in which medical staff offered little emotional support and then engaged in surgical, analgesic and medical intervention. Women frequently complained that their previous obstetricians explained the multiple risks associated with vaginal birth and suggested that C-section was statistically safer for babies. The myth of medicalised birth was fuelled from two directions: women's mistrust and dislike of medicalised birth; and the biomedical model that understands medicalised birth to be safer because it is the only legitimate, evidence based, 'true' means of practicing health care.

A doctor about to assist a C-section in a midwife-led birth jokingly remarked to Anouk 'never send a woman to do a man's job', implying that she had made the wrong choice in selecting a midwife to attend the birth. It also implied that Anouk could not actually birth her baby without (male) medical intervention. Women repeatedly reported how when they asked about using a midwife, their obstetrician made it clear that it was less safe and the safest choice was a C-section because the statistics suggest that infant mortality is slightly lower with C-sections than with vaginal births. In countering these arguments, midwives increasingly made recourse to the model of evidence-based practice, arguing that the latest literature on birth supported vaginal, non-surgical, unmedicated birth. (Note how it was medical evidence they were using to support their case, blurring the boundaries and distinctions between 'medical' and 'natural' birth; medical knowledge is used to bolster a claim for natural birth.) Yet, it appeared the perception that midwives were 'witch women', unable to be trusted, dangerous and risk-taking, was still felt by those adhering to the technocratic South African birth model (Cosslett 1994). Midwives spent much time explaining how a home birth was as safe as a hospital birth given that they carried all the equipment needed to resuscitate, stop bleeding and stabilise women and babies who were unconscious. Should a transfer to hospital become necessary, surgery or intervention would be available in approximately thirty minutes, whether in hospital or on the way, given that obstetricians and anaesthetists would need calling. As Beth said: 'a home birth is no different from an MOU birth – there is no theatre in the MOUs and women are transferred if problems arise, so birthing at home is birthing like most women in the Western Cape'. Despite this, women frequently described how friends and family saw their desire to home birth as irresponsible and dangerous, to the point that the women stopped speaking about it.

The hegemony of biomedicine has been powerful, but its reputation as a practice that forgoes nuances and alternate ways of knowing has been perhaps even more so. This was despite the fact that many doctors were caring, particularly the obstetricians who backed up the midwives, and many women who birthed in hospital remarked on how they liked the postpartum support staff (indeed, during my fieldwork I only heard one woman complain in a postnatal consultation about the hospital staff). Each midwife valued the role of epidural, ventouse or induction in particular contexts, yet the overarching perception that women who had medicalised birth would 'end up on their backs, under spot lights' remained firm. Absent from this perception was an acknowledgement that the back-up doctors all supported vaginal delivery and non-medicated pain relief practices (such as hypnobirthing, explained later, and breathing techniques) and many doctors in the Western Cape did support midwives and vaginal delivery but operated from hospitals that did not do so.[3]

Likewise, the ways in which biomedicine has impacted birth positively were not readily part of conversations, other than a cursory 'I'm glad C-sections exist for emergencies': after all, C-sections became a surgical practice to save the lives of women and babies where vaginal birth was not possible. Placenta praevia (where the placenta covers the cervix), true cephalopelvic disproportion (where the baby's head does not fit through the pelvis) and some breech positions, to name a few, are conditions that can require surgical intervention. The nuances, inflections and subtleties that often emerge when generalisations are abandoned went unacknowledged by most women using midwives. Yet, women still readily made use of 'medicalised' procedures when these ensured their safety. Grace was using the midwives for her second birth. She had a VBAC, after the delivery of her twins and spoke about the contrast between her births. Describing her decision to have a C-section to birth the twins, she said:

> My friend was with the Cape Town Midwives and pro-natural, and even she, she'd had her baby just before I had my twins, even she said I would definitely go caesarean with twins just because there are so many things [to go wrong]. So what often happens is the first twin is born naturally and then it's a complicated caesarean 'cos the one placenta might still be inside and then one is born naturally and one is caesarean and I didn't want that and I suppose there were all the possible complications.

Grace described her C-section experience:

> You're in a line up. Luckily I was first for the day but we're all sitting there, lambs to the slaughter, so there were a lot of things about it that I found disempowering and interestingly, what I can say now, throughout my whole pregnancy, was more disempowering because you're in the hands of a surgeon who is going to slice you open and take your baby out. When you know you're going natural, even if you end up having a Caesar, when you try for natural, your intention is natural and its 'hey little guy, you and I have to do this thing together, I hope you're lying right', you're visualising, you're reading, you're visualising him lying right and how he is going to be, and how you're going to be throughout your pregnancy, whereas with a caesarean section, it's like they're going to slice and take him out so I have no part in that actually, just got to lie still. For the natural, what was amazing was it was me, James (partner) and my midwives Tanya, that was it, Maggie was there at the start, the gynae was on standby cos it was a VBAC. She was at the door at one point, spoke to Tanya but didn't even step into the room. So it was just us which was amazing because with the twins, there were so many people in the room. There are 2 gynaes, an anaesthetist, a paediatrician, 4 nurses, any more? There's up to 8-10 people in the room apart from your husband and you and its very clinical and its very much a procedure and its very bright lights and I reacted to morphine, that was one of my biggest things so I felt zoned out, woozy and vomity, so when they tried to put my babies on me, it was just, 'get them away from me', I can't do this and then they just whip them off you and into

> bright lights and table and you know, manhandle them – they're just used to doing baby after baby after baby.

I describe her second birth in the next chapter. Grace set up a stark contrast between the two versions of birth: one of disempowerment, bright lights and feeling ill; the other, a room of quiet privacy and connection to her baby. Grace was able to use medicalised birth to ensure the safe delivery of her twins and felt that both kinds of birth had their place, but she did not recognise how different kinds of birth play out within one birthing model and the overlaps. She also did not factor in reactions to medication as part of what shaped her experience. The 'bright lights' and the large number of people in the operating theatre were blamed as part of the problems with medicalised birth and the reaction to medication and stress of the situation did not feature as elements that produced Grace's negative experience.[4]

Like Grace, many women described their birth experience as negative because it was medicalised, not noting that there were many elements at play in the production of a birth experience; these often went un-noted. Despite not all doctors being 'technocratic' in their orientation towards birth, they were still reviled and set up as diametrically opposed to 'natural' births and midwives. Institutional parameters, litigious orientations to adverse birth outcomes and convenience were factors that affected many South African women's 'choice' to have medicalised births, and medicalised and paternalistic doctors carried the blame for 'overly medicalised birth' in South Africa.

It is worth noting that people were more readily reviled than institutions in this scenario. Perhaps this is because many women in my study had private midwives present at hospital births and so for women like Grace, their birth experience was only able to be differentiated by who was there, not where they were. The hospital as a symbol of medicalised birth was filtered out of definitions of 'natural' birth and instead, the issue of who attended the birth was foregrounded. Yet it was the 'bright lights' and spatial issues that were cited as the reasons for not enjoying medicalised birth. It was also spatiality that in many ways defined a 'medicalised' birth, yet the fact that midwives trained and practiced in hospitals unsettles the boundaries of birth models.

Cultural storylines were in place as women contrasted versions of birth but the way in which women spoke about birth and the narratives they drew on did not reflect their actions, and their experiences undermined their narratives. As Grace 'chose' a C-section for a high-risk twin birth, she was making use of medicalised birth, yet she cited space as being the negative element of her experience. When Grace birthed 'naturally' she did so in hospital and yet the fact that both births were in a medicalised space did not feature in her differentiation of the births. The private midwives allowed for low lighting and no extra people were necessary; they did not require bright lights or extra assistance to perform surgery for Grace's VBAC. Therefore, even though Grace had a definite idea and differentiated two ideas of birth, how she actually differentiated them is not all that clear and her ideas of connection to the baby and fewer people in the room are not considered in relation to other factors, such as reacting to stress, the necessary requirements of surgery (lights and extra people) and analgesia.

The organising structure of a myth of birth is made complex by the players in birth decisions. While women framed their decisions as their 'own', there were multiple players who influenced their 'choices', besides 'pressurising' doctors. Partners, friends and colleagues recounted opinions and experiences of birth. People, institutions and views on birth were neatly differentiated in terms of medicalised and 'natural' birth but the differences were made blurry not only by overlaps in practices, but also by people in pregnant women's lives.

Complexities are evident in how Grace went about 'choosing' her C-section during her first pregnancy. There are several players that come to bear on women's decision making. Even though Grace framed it as her 'own' 'choice', it was actually her friend and other social pressures and factors that put her off attempting a vaginal birth the first time round (even though of course twin vaginal births do happen) knowing the risks of 'natural' twin delivery. Grace's doctor on the other hand would have been legally required to explain birthing options and the risks associated with each, although she does not offer the doctor's view in her account. Yet in Grace's view, the blame for how she experienced her first birth was laid on her doctors, the medical system and ideas of medicalised birth. Concurrently, 'natural' birth for twins was framed as risky by Grace's friends, family and colleagues but it was the medical system that supposedly 'forces', 'cajoles' and 'pressures' women into surgical births by stating the dangers and risks of 'natural' birth; other social pressures that might lead women to 'choose' a natural birth are discounted. Yet the pressure from doctors was a common theme. This was a sentiment that was reflected by the midwives.

The midwives set themselves against medicalised birth on the basis that they offered one-to-one care, continuous labour support, and a quiet space and calm environment in which to birth. Maggie told Michaela:

> You will hear voices, noises, sounds and expressions you have never heard from yourself. You will see another side of yourself, it's primal and if you can, it's the best thing to ever do, have a natural birth. As labour progresses it's like changing gear, you move to the next stage with different techniques and that often women are stronger than they think. It's nice to have a midwife right through because the doctors coming in when it's time to push, at the end, are often a bit scared seeing the woman in full, active labour whereas if we're with you throughout, we've seen you develop over the course of the labour and we're used to it by then.

To some degree the contrast was true: medical doctors did not support women by being present right through labour. However, this does not mean that when they were there, the care was not supportive or encouraging of the atmosphere women wanted, nor did it mean that doctors were 'scared', a somewhat exaggerated descriptor.

Women in South Africa using midwives drew on US narratives such as Ina May Gaskin's *Spiritual Midwifery* and Marie Mongan's *Hypnobirthing*, two books frequently recommended by the midwives, as 'evidence' of the cruelties and injustices of medicalised births. Mongan wrote of her own experiences birthing in hospital. She described being strapped down, unable to move, administered analgesia, with forceps being used to 'rip' the baby from a woman's body. Medical births were described using language sets that included words like 'rip', 'cut' and 'slice'. This language suggests a loss of control of women's bodies as babies are 'ripped' from them and they are 'sliced' open.

A language of violence and trauma is used to account for (i.e. is presented as fact) how women said they experienced birth, but also how language was naturalised and came to inflect perceptions that medicalised birth was automatically and intrinsically traumatic. During my conversations with them, midwives frequently described doctors as medical professionals trained for risk management whereas midwives were 'specialists in normal birth'. Using words such as violence and trauma, Kitzinger (1992), Oakley (1980), Martin (1987), Humphreys (1998) and Maclean, McDermott and May (2000) suggest that the medicalised birth model violates women, leaving them with trauma, stress and fear because the control of birth and its associated practices, such as decisions on whether to have induction and forceps, are in the hands of medical professionals not labouring women.

These feelings, while extreme, were expressed mainly by women having VBACs in consultations, who had used an obstetrician for their first birth, and who stated that they had been so traumatised they had transferred to a midwife for their subsequent births. However, it should be noted that the midwives did not have many clients having VBACs given that the obstetrician was usually the primary carer for a woman attempting a VBAC, with midwives playing a supportive rather than directive role. Out of 220 women that were cared for by the midwives where I was present, eighteen spoke of trauma personally or described the need to change to a midwife after hearing about a friend's traumatic experience. This accounts for 8.2 per cent of the women in the study.

Oakley (1980), Martin (1987), Humphreys (1998) and Maclean, McDermott and May (2000) have all written to expose the distressing quality of some medicalised births, but as Chadwick (2007: 44) points out, the problem with the 'fight for natural birth' model is that it places women as entirely passive to the practices and effects of medicalised birth: women have been led to believe that their bodies cannot birth and that medicalised birth is safer, with women metaphorically leaving the picture of birth altogether. Bearing in mind that women still die in childbirth and that basic care is still unavailable for certain women, specifically in South Africa where women at MOUs do not have the option of an epidural or a constant carer, the narrative of a 'fight' for natural birth is specific to middle-class women of a particular socio-economic status and race (Chadwick 2007).[5]

Chadwick (2007) notes that Katz Rothman (1982) and Davis-Floyd (1992) both offer inadequate accounts of 'natural' birth (midwife or holistic birth). She argues that births are framed within patriarchal terms and thus ideas of differentiated models of birth, even a so-called natural model, are not outside patriarchal discourse. The two models are therefore connected and attempting to subvert patriarchy in birthing talk is not as easy as it is presented by Katz Rothman and David-Floyd. I argue, drawing from and building on Cosslett (1994), that this is because 'natural' birth cannot be defined outside of contrasts with medicalised birth. 'Natural' and 'medicalised' birth exist as one another's other. These storylines included the perception of medicalised safety in surgical and medical intervention, along with the perception of the cold, clinical, careless quality of biomedicine. Yet both understandings were a myth: a myth that the biomedical model is right, objective and absolute, and so too, the perception of the cold, carelessness of medicalised birth. The critiques of biomedicine have shown that it is not absolute as a health practice and the subtleties and personal qualities of medical doctors are obscured in the stereotype of a clinical, uncaring interaction. We shall see though that these perceptions played a role in how birthing relations were made and the kinds of attentions women desired.

The Natural Birth Myth

When I began speaking with midwives and their clients about why women chose to have midwife-led births it was clear that women and midwives saw 'intervention-free' birth as the most desirable form of birth, if possible. It was only once I began the hypnobirthing class, a birth preparation class that combines hypnosis with relaxation techniques for helping women work through labour, that the history and underpinnings of the natural childbirth movement became clear, informing the ideas of some women seeking a particular version of birth in South Africa.

The story of the natural birth movement began in 1913 (as opposed to the anthropological and feminist concerns with medical birth in the 1970s), when Grantly Dick-Read, an intern, was called to attend to a women in labour in London's East End. He arrived and immediately offered the woman chloroform (the standard analgesia in that period), but she refused. Dick-Read observed the birth and watched as the woman quietly birthed her baby. Afterwards, Dick-Read asked why the woman did not want pain relief. She replied: 'it didn't hurt. It wasn't supposed to, was it, doctor?' Following his East End experience, Dick-Read encountered births supposedly in World War I (where he encountered women in war is unclear) where women in labour were directed to Dick-Read but never asked for assistance, just the assurance that he was nearby. Each of these women birthed with what appeared to be great ease and no pain, quickly birthing, wrapping up their babies and heading on to their destination. Dick-Read was confused by what he saw in the rural village settings compared to the agony middle-class women appeared to experience in hospital, a setting where nurses spoke of 'boring' work nights when there were no 'problem' births.

Dick-Read pondered his observations and came to the conclusion that for the 'simple', working-class women, the absence of fear was what separated their births from those of middle-class women in hospital and so began Dick-Read's theory that fear produced pain (Dick-Read did not appear to factor in that working-class women generally did more physical labour throughout the day which could have accounted for these differences). In this model, fear caused the arteries to the uterus to constrict, allowing less blood flow and a constricted, tense uterus rather than a relaxed, open uterus that easily expels a baby. Dick-Read called this the fear-tension-pain syndrome, and published his findings in *Childbirth without Fear* (1933). While his theories were rejected at the time because they were understood to hold no scientific validity as there was no knowledge of hormones in birth, Marie Mongan, author of *Hypnobirthing* (1992), notes that in the 1970s, the sciences discovered the work of endorphins and oxytocin as 'the body's natural pain killers'. As the main contributor on the importance of oxytocin, Michel Odent (1984), a French obstetrician, began writing on the effects of intervention in birth, a process that he suggests, when left to being entirely physiological and not disturbed by medical intervention and other people (for Odent women should birth alone where they feel safe), is pain-free and productive. Odent (wombecology.com) writes:

> Long before the industrialisation of childbirth, all cultures have disturbed the birth process and therefore the in-labour intrauterine environment, even if only through beliefs and rituals. This is why we must first refer to the physiological perspective. Physiologists look at what is universal and cross-cultural. They offer a sort of reference point. Then the effects of the most common deviations from the physiological reference will be more easily interpreted.
>
> All mammals give birth thanks to the sudden release of a flow of hormones. One of these hormones – namely oxytocin – plays a pivotal role. It is necessary to contract the uterus for the birth of the babies and for the delivery of the placentas. It is involved in the induction of maternal love: it is the main component of a real 'cocktail of love hormones' (among the other components of this cocktail are endorphins, prolactin, and vasopressin). All mammals can also release an emergency hormone – namely adrenaline – whose effect is to stop the release of oxytocin. The emergency hormone adrenaline is released in particular when there is a possible danger.
>
> The fact that adrenaline and oxytocin are antagonistic explains that the basic need of all mammals giving birth is to feel secure. In a wild

> environment a female cannot give birth as long as there is a possible danger, for example the presence of a predator around. In that case it is an advantage to release adrenaline, which brings more blood to the skeletal muscles and gives more energy to fight or to run away; it is also an advantage to stop releasing oxytocin and to postpone the birth process. Mammals release adrenaline when they feel observed. It is noticeable that they all rely on a specific strategy not to feel observed when giving birth: privacy is obviously another basic need. The emergency hormone is also involved in thermoregulation. In a cold environment one of the well-known roles of adrenaline is to induce the process of vasoconstriction.

Odent sets up a division between nature and culture in which birth is physiological and any social element in birth is cultural. He fails to acknowledge that his analysis and studies on birth are entrenched in scientific forms of knowledge, as cultural practice. He works from the assumption that all that science deemed optimal for birth, without surgical interventions or medications, is natural. This establishes a myth of birth. His model prioritises physiology; it is premised on a notion that all bodies, everywhere, are the same. His model draws on notions of the primal body that underpins the nature/culture divide: a body that is universal and outside the influence of culture. As I have shown, Lock and Nguyen (2010) present a model of bodies as neither fixed nor universal and produced in relation to social and cultural life. Yet Odent's framing of bodies and birth is powerful.

On multiple occasions during fieldwork I was told that birthing was analogous to a deer in the wild. Should there be any stress, in the form of noise, too many people, and bright lights, like a deer sensing danger, adrenaline would be released, labour would stop and the deer would run away to safety. Rather than being offended by an analogy likening women to deer, women revelled in it, enjoying the idea of birthing 'as nature intended' and how birth is 'primitively, in the wild'. Likewise, women imagined themselves birthing like the frequently imagined and generalised, though never specified, rural black woman who would feel labour, breathe deeply and squat behind a wall, birthing her baby, wrapping it on her back, before going back to work in the fields. Women were drawing on a combination of a romanticised past and a scientific understanding of birth where knowledge of hormones and the physiological process of birth were necessary.

The practice of theorising 'natural' birth is a cultural practice and an intervention, as is a knowledge of hormones and their impact on the body and labour. Imaginings of the wild and all that belongs to 'nature' have a long history in the modernist project that emphasised the separation of nature and culture, in which science is framed as the source of objective knowledge about nature. Women using midwives, as well as midwives themselves, framed their reasoning for wanting and promoting the desired, vaginal birth as 'natural' because science had deemed it the means by which women birth, and scientific studies had proved the benefits of that form of birth. That labour and birth are physiological events that sometimes do not work and result in death or the need for medical intervention were factored out of the understandings of 'natural birth'. Practically speaking though, the midwives told women they had to work to get the birth they wanted and understood the risks of birth and tried to manage women's expectations of birth: it does not always go as one plans. The overarching narrative of birth was that it was natural and this was confirmed by the objectivity of science.

Yet it was cultural storylines of the truth of science that had produced the medicalised, technocratic versions of birth that women and their midwives understood themselves to be working against. Despite the consistent framing that medical intervention had its place when necessary with 'safety coming first', the overriding discourse was one where women wanted to birth as 'nature intended' and midwives sought to support women in their right to birth as they wanted, providing them with the means to do so as carers. Rights and choice were woven together as women engaged with pregnancy and labour care as consumers. Rather than framing safe care as a human right, the kinds of care and birth instantiated by midwives were foregrounded. In reality though, midwives used medical intervention, births went awry and midwives were indeed an intervention, offering support and help in positioning the baby. In these representations, risk and safety, while spoken about, did not have to be a primary worry: women 'knew' their midwives had the skill and equipment to deal with a risky situation. The midwives tended to and practised the safety parameters and knowledge of safety that women wanted. Those parameters and knowledge allowed women to 'choose' how to birth outside of questions of risk and in making that choice, even though safety was one of the factors, it did not have to be the main one. How one birthed did not need to be thought through in terms of safety as the midwives covered this, trusted as biomedical professionals and backed up by biomedical specialists. The language of birth, and birth as a limit condition (a temporary period, although one that was framed as normal in the midwifery model) was not framed in safety terms. Thus an interesting melding of birthing models of language played out as midwives attempted to normalise an event that is both hard work and for some women, particularly in sub-Saharan Africa, dangerous. 'Choice' in how women wanted to birth overrode 'choice' in terms of birthing safety and risk because these did not need to be considered. Medical back-up and support largely ensured safe delivery.

To Be One Another's Other

Midwives offered hands-on continuity of care with a 'conducive' birthing environment. Neither they nor their clients understood those practices as forms of intervention. Indeed, neither does most of the birthing literature (see Kitzinger 1962, Davis-Floyd 1992, Chadwick 2007). Both renditions of what I have described as myths employed science and both used different versions of knowledge to provide arguments for why one version of birth was better than another.

The birth scene encountered in middle-class private health care was not about knowledge and alternate ways of knowing. It was about two myths, dependent on one another, and both premised on and within science that determined a particular discourse. There are also considerable resonances with the ways in which 'choices' are presented and made in contemporary consumer culture. While my data do not necessarily back the contention made by Katz Rothman (1982) and Treichler (1990) that birthing is subject to the same pressures as those that drive commodification and consumption, it is worth noting that the terms in which people express their desires rest on consumerist framings – choice, entitlement and service. These factors came to make choice the axis upon which birth was approached by South African middle-class women seeking care in the private sector.

The nature/culture divide separating the versions of birth possible is premised on science's modernist project. As I have shown, South Africa's colonial history, which opposed 'tradition', 'the rural', 'the primitive' to 'the rational', controlled and sterile, formed the basis for who birthed in homes with midwives or laywomen and who did so in hospitals with doctors. In today's context, those histories live on: it is mainly middle-class women with access to medical insurance who birth via elective C-section in hospitals.

More specifically, it is largely white, middle-class women who have been able to frame birth within a discourse of choice. The biomedical training of midwives, the parameters of safety and the ready availability of medical and surgical intervention when needed are the specific reasons why 'choosing' how to birth is possible. It is also why middle-class women usually experience safe delivery despite living in a region where infant mortality is high. Privilege is choice for these women. Privilege is also having a safety net that can be taken for granted.

Indeed, the women in my study did not talk about birth risk often and there is a critical reason for this. It is necessary to acknowledge the argument that middle-class women are distanced from issues of life and death. Life is not precarious and because of medical insurance, women in my study did not need to worry about being cared for medically in birth or any other medical necessity. This fact is central to the imaginings of the wrongs of 'technocratic' birth due to the availability of medical back-up; this back-up is taken for granted, as a given. This back-up (that is a 'given') allows women to frame birth in particular ways – as safe because it is 'natural' – as they are able to rely on back-up support without the concern or worry that it might not be available. Being able to birth 'naturally' and safely is a luxury. This is critical to the imagining of both 'natural' birth and 'women's work'.

The Work of Myth

In *The Effectiveness of Symbols* (1963), Levi-Strauss describes the rare occurrence of a Cuna woman in Panama struggling through a difficult childbirth. The shaman is summoned to attend the birth while the midwife continues trying to assist the baby. An incantation, consisting of 535 sections transcribed over eighteen pages, describes the process of the birth – how the midwife is confused, her visits to the shaman, his arrival and preparations of burning cocoa nibs, the calling on spirits for assistance via wood carvings and invocations. The incantation then moves to the finding of the 'soul' of the labouring woman, which has been stolen by *Muu*, the force that produces life: a difficult birth results when *Muu* exceeds her power. This is a story of the shaman engaging in a brave journey to the mythical spiritual realm in order to find the labouring woman's lost 'double'. The woman's uterus becomes a world in which fantastical creatures are battled by the shaman, manifested in her pains and discomfort. The shaman's work ends with the safe delivery of the baby. All the while, the shaman never touches the woman: the 'cure' is entirely verbal.

Levi-Strauss (1963: 192) argues that the incantation and ritual serve to invoke a psychological manipulation for a physiological cure. Moving between the mythical and physiological, more rapidly, having journeyed the woman through the narrative of evil and good forces and the process of summoning the shaman, via the incantation, the difference between the mythological and physiological, through speech, is blurred and the mythical process of opening her to retrieve her spirit provides the symbolic opening to helping her physiology, to effect a safe delivery. Levi-Strauss writes:

> The cure would consist, therefore, in making explicit a situation originally existing on the emotional level and in rendering acceptable to the mind pains which the body refuses to tolerate. That the mythology of the shaman does not correspond to an objective reality does not matter... The sick woman accepts these mythical beings or, more accurately, she has never questioned their existence.

For middle-class women in South Africa, like the Cuna woman, the fact that the myth of birth did not correspond with reality and experience did not, in some ways, matter. Having the option of two different versions of birth produced and was part of a consumer-driven approach to birthing and that created a 'choice'. The inflections of different waves of feminist discourse separating versions of birth and who controlled birth, the political economy of doctors and women choosing surgical births for convenience and litigious orientations to risk came to bear on the maintenance and organisation of a myth that allowed women to approach their births as individuals making choices. The implications of this include birthing care as a service and as Davis-Floyd (1994) notes, choice in birth, particularly technocratic birth, being empowering.

In other ways though it is not empowering and 'choice' implies control. Despite the myth and the imaginary of choice, experience showed that birth cannot be controlled and planning does not guarantee a desired outcome. A set of effects emerged alongside the framing of birth as a choice: 'natural' births were achievements and by extension, surgical and 'medicalised' births were failures. This is a devastating consequence.

Here, the work of midwives and the midwives themselves as interventions is critical but slipped from view. The hard work of producing a desired version of birth by midwives was made invisible beneath the myth of 'natural' birth under the guise of 'it worked because it's natural'. The work of myth was made clear: it changed how women engaged with birth as a 'choice' in how they used their bodies in life-giving work and it shifted how midwives were imagined, flattening the effects one person and their body had on another's version of birth, the ways in which bodies materialised and how women thought through birth experiences and their bodies. They were able to do so because they had 'options', and as a result, particular kinds of planning, approaches and care emerged in relation to a model of birth.

Notes

1. Midwives had medical insurance like the obstetricians who backed them up, but midwives' insurance was far less than obstetric medical insurance.
2. These were argued by Katz Rothman (1982), in her 'midwifery model', and Davis-Floyd (1992), in her 'holistic model', to be partnership-orientated births using midwives and family as core carers and supporters of birth.
3. Private sector hospitals in South Africa are privately owned and therefore have their own rules and regulations. Doctors rent rooms from hospitals and therefore have to practise under hospital management and according to their rules to a large degree. As a private institution, hospitals are vulnerable to a litigation orientated client base and therefore hospital management establishes parameters understood to reduce risk and law suits by banning independent midwives while employing midwives in-house.
4. Not all women have bad reactions to analgesia and thus feeling ill was not an inevitable experience of 'medicalised' birth.
5. Maternal Mortality Rates for South Africa are 625 per 100,000 women (MDG 2000).

Chapter 2

Being Heard

Planning, 'Choice' and Knowing in Pregnancy and Birth

The women in my study held particular definitions of natural birth and they approached elite birthing care as consumers. Natural birth had come to stand as a contrasting model to medicalised, surgical birth for the women with whom I worked, thus the myth-making process of birth established a context in which choosing to birth between competing models was at stake. Birthing care was offered as a service for this group of women; they saw birth as a choice-based practice to be controlled and they approached their pregnancies as plan.[1] When using the term and concept of 'pregnancy as plan', I mean that the women in my study understood their pregnancies as 'projects' and they tried to plan how, when and with whom elements of their pregnancies would unfold. I use Orit Avishai's (2007) idea of motherhood as a project, an experience that can entail planning and management, to elaborate on themes of knowing, risk and trust.[2] The pregnancy as plan approach required knowledge of the kinds of birth available and how to 'do it'. Here, I look closely at the ways in which midwives and their clients engaged one another and how different ways of knowing, informing, engaging and negotiating are constituted and differentiated as a reproductive event was framed as a project by middle-class women (Avishai 2007). In doing so, I demonstrate how being able to plan and educate oneself on how one births reflects an easily taken for granted privilege (as choice and availability of knowledge). As I will show, woman sought a mode of recognition, to be seen in certain ways; theirs was not an experience of survival, but acknowledgment.

Margaret MacDonald (2007) suggests that choice is integral to midwifery-led care. By this she means that midwives in Canada (although it applies to South Africa too, given that midwifery models of care travel) believed in providing the pros and cons of birthing procedures and practices. Offering pros and cons is not unique to the midwifery model but is emphasised as such. An informed choice model emerges within midwifery care as midwives placed importance on explaining details and allowing personal experience to be accounted for in women's decision-making processes. In other words, intuition and experience are given as much value as more 'rational' ways of knowing (MacDonald 2007: 101). The idea of choice is part of being modern. Being able to be concerned by planning and choices is not universal in the South African context. Heather Paxson (2002: 308) suggests that there are varying ways in which people classify themselves and are defined as modern – family size, reproductive strategies and gender roles are some of the dialogues that offer spaces for people to navigate ideas of modernity. Medical technology, contraception and birthing options form part of the modernisation project. In her study, Paxson (2004) reveals that good, modern women are understood to exercise rationality, responsibility and choice. Having choice and exercising good choices is part of being modern (and privileged). Having choices is to some degree expected of women (Paxson 2002). Therefore, MacDonald argues that having knowledge and a sense of control – choice – is integral in defining (and I would add having) a natural birth experience.

In the South African context, the relationship between being 'a modern person' and having choice holds but having women as consumers adds another dimension to how South African middle-class women engaged with choices in birthing. I argue that because women were educated, constituted part of an elite economic bracket and were paying for the service of birthing care, pregnancy was engaged as plan. Notions of choice, informed choice, a right to choose and being recognised as a rights-holding, paying client shaped how women with whom I interacted approached their pregnancies and sought to know their bodies. A project of good mothering, a standard set for economically elite women who consult expert advice and research reproductive work, was at stake

(Avishai 2007). Indeed, Avishai (2007) argues that the embodied experience anticipated in reproductive work can be overwhelming. Managing breastfeeding, pregnancy and birth as projects can make this work seem less overwhelming. Extending the notion of reproductive work as a project, I argue that the pregnancy as plan acted as a mode for allowing women to be seen and heard in particular ways: women who were seen to be enacting the universal feminine work of birthing and becoming, as a result, good mothers. As women came to know and manage pregnancy in certain ways, their midwives responded. These ways of responding constituted several modes of attentiveness. The chapter engages with questions on the relationship between 'informed' choice, knowing and planning and the place of education, knowledge, privilege and solace in modern maternal care practices.

Ways of Knowing and Practices of Making Plans around Pregnancy

Tina was thirty weeks pregnant when we met at one of the birth preparation classes (see Chapter 3) that I attended in the first few months of fieldwork. She was accompanied by her friend and had chosen to become pregnant through sperm donation (she was one amongst five women who became pregnant this way over the course of my study). As we introduced ourselves to one another, Tina explained that aside from wanting a 'natural' birth, she had a blood disorder that made the use of analgesia inadvisable. She wanted to have tools in place to help her get through birth unmedicated. In an interview I conducted with her after the birth of her daughter, she described how, quite apart from her medical condition, she had 'always liked the idea of natural', adding 'it's how babies are meant to be born'. 'Women's bodies are designed to birth vaginally' she explained. This came to be a common phrase during fieldwork. In Tina's case it is clear that a flexible engagement with the definitions and modulating of the term 'natural' existed. Despite having a medical condition, birthing under enormous supervision was still a 'natural' birth. For Tina, her birth would still be 'natural' because it was vaginal, without the use of analgesia or induction and she was birthing with the support of midwives, who would make decisions with her.

Tina was the only woman in the class who had chosen not to know the sex of her baby. She did not mind 'what she had', she was 'just happy to be having a baby'. I was particularly struck by Tina's insistence on a 'natural' birth given her 'non-natural' route to becoming pregnant. Clearly, like her medical condition, Tina's use of artificial insemination (AI) did not interrupt her understanding of and desire for a 'natural' birth. Tina, like many other women, constructed and chose a version of what natural birth meant to her and how it was defined. Unmedicated vaginal delivery was critical to her sense of herself as a good mother. She did not see her desire to have a 'natural' birth as contradictory given how she became pregnant. The medicalised techniques of conception and delivery were separated in her mind. For her, birth preparation tools fell within the parameters of natural birth, medicated birth did not. It appeared that the birth itself was more important in constituting ideas of 'natural' than the methods for becoming pregnant or 'preparing' for birth.

Over the next five weeks, Tina learned about both the physiology and emotional dimensions of labour. She learned about both oxytocin and the importance of 'letting go of fears around birth'. Instructors taught her how she could use visualisation and breathing techniques to help offset the pain of birth. She was anxious about the potential for needing analgesia and having heard about how painful birth was from colleagues, friends and passers-by, found the positive atmosphere of classes a refreshing change from what she had grown used to hearing. As time passed, Tina began to speak about who would attend her birth: her friend and the midwife, the back-up obstetrician and her mother. As I listened to her in the class's tea breaks, Tina began to imagine and craft a hospital-based birthing space that was private and, despite her medical condition, as 'non-medicalised' as possible. Her new knowledge of birth became part of a set of arrangements that determined how, where and with whom Tina would birth. As a mothering project, the space and attendants were key in planning her birth and even though she needed to be in hospital, the midwife-led birth provided an avenue for 'informed choice' and 'natural birth'.

Two weeks after the classes ended, I saw Tina for her thirty-eight-week consultation with one of the Cape Town midwives, Tanya. Tina came into the consultation appearing slightly rushed and flustered: she was speaking quickly and began talking immediately about the pregnancy with no 'small talk'. She explained her worries about how her sciatica was 'playing up' and the multiple tests she had had to check on her condition. Tanya laughed when Tina said 'I'm going into this birth like a normal person' because they had spoken about clotting factors and the effects of medication: a lot more 'medical' conversation than most 'normal' pregnancies entailed. They also spoke about how Ingrid, another midwife in the practice, had done plenty of research on the condition for the rest of the team and knew Tina better than the other midwives despite not having met her yet. Tanya assured Tina that she was sure her body would do 'exactly as it should' and when doing the physical check, Tanya spoke to Tina's baby asking 'how are you today?' Tina visibly relaxed, her shoulders lowered, she smiled and spoke more slowly and said that she could go into the birth without fear, trusting her midwives knew about her situation and how to care for her.

The rhythm of the consultation, half an hour long, had gone from fast-paced to slow; from anxious and flustered, it settled on the joy of anticipating birth. A large portion of the consultation had been devoted to discussing biomedical procedures and Tina's medical condition but she still considered herself 'normal' and able to birth naturally. The sets of language and the ways of talking medically were offset by Tanya's assurance that Tina's body could be trusted, which shifted the tone and rhythm of the consultation. The midwife produced and marked the 'feeling' of natural birth: calm reassurances and focusing on the baby. Tina's concern and management of her pregnancy was overshadowed by her broader planning in which she had chosen a midwife-led birth. Normalising pregnancy was at the core of the midwifery care model. Thus, Tina's carer focused attention on the baby and Tina's body: a body able to birth. The fact that Tina needed to be reassured of her body's capacity to birth suggests the broader apparatus that shapes women's experiences of their bodies, in which alienation is at the centre. Avishai (2007: 136) argues that making mothering a project offers women an avenue for engaging with 'a threatening, alien and otherwise unintelligible embodied practice'. The question of why Tina needed a carer who affirmed her body's ability is partly answered by the framework of dichotomised models of birth in which natural birth has been set up as the antidote to women's lack of control in and ability to birth (Kitzinger 1992, Katz Rothman 1982) as well as the difficulty of approaching, for the first time, an extreme, bodily event. By choosing a midwife, Tina was doing work in which she shaped her experience and was engaging with a carer who positioned her as a woman able to birth.

A week later, Tina came into her consultation, this time with midwife Ingrid, whom she had not yet met, but who had informed herself and the midwifery team about Tina's condition. They began speaking as if they had had a prior conversation and were picking up where they left off (indeed Tina had spoken to one of the midwives the day before when her waters broke and the other midwives had been made aware of Tina's early rupturing of membranes). Tina had been running errands and picking up last minute baby items at the pharmacy when she had felt a small rush of liquid and thought she had wet herself: her waters had broken. Ruptured membranes at thirty-eight weeks was not in itself problematic but Tina had yet to go into labour and risk of infection would increase should she not deliver in the next few days. A C-section was becoming more likely.

Tina was upset about what had transpired. Her friend, who had accompanied her to the consultation, commented that she had had such 'an easy time' up until now, adding that it was a pity that her 'plans were unravelling'. Ingrid sat Tina on the examining table to check her blood pressure and the baby's wellbeing. Tina cried throughout the examination. She was upset about the increased probability of a C-section along with the distressing experience of suddenly, uncontrollably, feeling liquid pour out of her body every so often (once there is a rupturing, amniotic fluid can intermittently continue to leak) and the weight of having to make a decision she did not want to make for the kind of birth she had planned carefully not to have. Tina sat with Ingrid, discussing her options: to be induced and try for vaginal birth which might not work, or go straight for an elective C-section so that if the induction did not work there would be no need to rush into surgery.

Tina asked Ingrid what she would do if she were in her situation. Ingrid said that all the options had their merits but did not offer her opinion; she asked Tina what she thought the options were and listened as she spoke about not wanting the stress and unpredictability of an emergency C-section and the importance of her own and her baby's safety along with as gentle a birth as possible. Without Ingrid's saying much, Tina decided she would book an 'elective' C-section even if she did not feel it was 'elective' given that she did not want it.[3] Ingrid smiled and told her it was not the end of the world, she was still going to have a baby and she had done well in making a decision.

After this consultation, Ingrid told me that she had thought Tina should be induced and try for a vaginal delivery, as she saw no reason why it would not work, but that she had sensed that Tina had seemed to 'want to go the C-section route' and so had supported her choice rather than offering an opinion or imposing her own judgment. In this instance, Ingrid chose to withhold information, engaging a 'sense' of her client's emotional state and factoring emotions into a decision about a physiological event.

Tina's language illustrates the extent to which women engaging midwives understood their births to be choices. It reveals the deep upset experienced when a pregnancy did not 'go to plan'. It also reveals the ways in which safety is assumed and its route (a C-section) is seen as an unfortunate outcome rather than a life-saving measure. The term 'elective' C-section has taken on a particular valence in South African birthing circles. It is often negatively valued and among women choosing midwife-assisted birth entailed a moralistic mode of thinking: an 'elective' C-section was seen as worse than an 'emergency' one. An 'emergency' C-section is seen as medically justified and therefore necessary; it is viewed as the only acceptable kind of medicalised intervention. An 'elective' C-section is portrayed as somehow being 'a cop out': a refusal to deal with the unruly and potentially painful procedures of birth and of womanhood. The negative valence is attached to understandings of both the deferral of power over one's body and birthing to a masculinised medical establishment and to a sanitised process that denies the power of the feminine. However, as is clear in the description above, the term 'elective' is elastic. For Tina, it was provocative because it brought attention to the unravelling lack of control she had in how she birthed, while at the same time simultaneously suggesting that it was 'her choice'; that is, locating her as the source of an option that is negatively valenced. Having to 'choose' an 'elective' C-section in a context in which she felt herself to be approaching an emergency went directly against her 'choice' to birth naturally. Notice here how the language of choice undermines the context in which decisions have to be made; Tina's birthing record would state that she had an elective C-section, not that she experienced the onset of birthing as a medical emergency and took proactive decisions to avert potential harm. It is worth noting that despite the undertones of 'elective' and 'emergency' for Tina, she actually chose a more medicalised route to birthing and saw that as the less 'risky' option. This is interesting given her emphasis on the importance of birthing vaginally as 'less risky' for her condition.

Tina made a decision that entailed navigating the valencing of words, adhering to particular notions of the 'natural' but simultaneously melding definitions in her route to pregnancy and choices around birth. Informed choice was shadowed by the obligation to plan and order life and engage modes for what Beck-Gernsheim (1996) calls 'preventative protection'. The ways in which people engage with ideas of choice in modern reproduction is layered according to tensions between constructions of the cyborg body – the fusing of machines, bodies and technologies – and modern bodies, the former figured around ideas of flexibility and choice, the latter by ideas of control. This is an intriguing notion in relation to the underpinnings of the universal feminine. The universal feminine draws on ideas of a primal femininity inherent to all women yet the cyborg body is framed around ideas of flexibility and choice – the notions considered to be the defining factors in natural birth and universal feminine work. In reproduction, emphasis is placed on control and as Paxson (2002) suggests, is part of being a modern woman. Yet simultaneously, reproductive technologies point to individual choices and plasticity in family formation (Clarke 1995, Franklin 1997). Indeed, when her waters broke 'early', Tina felt she had no choice at all but to opt for an 'elective' C-section that made invisible her planning for a natural birth. In fact, as it turned out Tina spontaneously went into labour that evening and she delivered her daughter 'naturally' after a slow labour.

When we met a few weeks after the birth, Tina described how she had found it hard to 'let go' when dilation was slow. She had become despondent. Tanya, the midwife in attendance at the birth, told her she thought she could 'do it' but an epidural would help move the labour along. Despite her anxieties around analgesia, Tina agreed to the epidural and the next morning when the doctor came to check on Tina and her unborn baby, Tanya asked for a few more hours before surgery. In that time Tina delivered her daughter. Tina was grateful to her midwives, feeling they had advocated for her when the pressure to birth in a certain number of hours was increasing. Tanya had offset time pressures as well as Tina's worry over the use of analgesia and Tina was able to birth for the most part as she had wanted. That desire was modified by the use of analgesia – that is, the birth she had was not the birth she planned – but the 'elective' C-section was averted and Tina was satisfied with her labour and delivery despite elements of medical intervention.

Pregnancy as a Project: Constituting the Planning and Knowing of Pregnancy

During Tina's pregnancy, she and her midwives engaged in ways that allowed Tina to feel that she was part of the decision-making process and the plans and definitions for her birth were modulated over the course of the pregnancy and during interactions with the midwives. As described above, Tina had told Tanya she did not need to fear birth because she trusted her midwives to handle the details of birth and her condition. On a second occasion I witnessed Ingrid withholding her opinion on how Tina should birth because she had felt that Tina had a preference and she needed to respect that. The third time happened in labour, as Tanya described the benefits of an epidural in certain cases, despite what Tina had learned and feared about medicated birth. The definition of natural birth shifted as events transpired. Whereas Tina had not originally categorised an epidural as part of the natural birth experience, her parameters changed. MacDonald (2007) calls this a flexible construction of natural birth and argues that this strengthens ideas of empowerment because it allows for a range of options that can be shaped to the emergent conditions of pregnancies. Indeed, Tina's plans had changed, but she felt she still had options and, significantly, she felt 'heard' as Tanya advocated for her and her wishes. The feeling of being heard is critical: Tina did not get the birth she had originally planned but she did feel that she was consulted in decision-making processes and her wishes were respected. Being heard is therefore a key theme in the kind of care being offered by midwives. Being heard is a mode of privilege and an experience that can be purchased as service. Elastic definitions of 'natural' birth are modulated and MacDonald (2007) points out that flexible constructions of birth strengthen notions of empowerment. Yet here it becomes clear that even ideas of empowerment can be modulated in accordance with birth models, models of care and flexible constructions of birth. Rather than presenting women with an 'either/or' scenario in ideas of empowerment, women like Tina felt empowered because they were heard. Tina's planning had situated her in a context where she would be listened to by her care providers. There were several ways in which she was therefore able to engage with knowledge and coming to know (about birth).

For instance, Tina negotiated different perspectives on pain depending on who she spoke to: hypnobirthing peers or her own peers and passers-by. The negotiations had played out between Tina, other people, popular knowledge and research on birth and its associated interventions, pregnancy and versions of birth, and between midwife and client. There were several layers to how Tina was informed and uninformed and how she deliberated on and made choices in pregnancy and birth. Her 'coming to know' – of her desires, her body and her research-informed vision – had multiple locations and was in line with Lock and Scheper-Hughes' (1987) suggestion that knowledge connected to the body is culturally constructed, reformed and renegotiated. The knowledge of how to birth was partly exteriorised, that is, it was part of Tina's plans and research, and was also assumed to be 'interior', located in her body as an 'innate ability' to birth. Some of her knowledge, or how much she learned was located in her knowing her midwives. Knowledge and its placement was malleable. Tina's story is illustrative of the ways in which choice, planning, knowing and risk coalesced. It demonstrates how Tina reformulated and negotiated definitions of natural birth and emphasises the place of choice. Tina's case points to several themes that emerged consistently among the women in my study. Issues of planning, research, evaluations of risk and flexible definitions are key to how they understood their roles and responsibilities during pregnancy. Knowing, being knowledgeable and engaging knowledge are central themes in middle-class women's experiences of pregnancy. Below, I demonstrate how women came to negotiate the ways in which they came to know pregnancy as a choice-based practice.

Decision Making, Knowing and Notions of Risk

Knowing is constituted in many ways. Sometimes knowing of a person (and what they might symbolise) is significant. Here, I unpack safety, knowing and planning in terms of knowing of the midwife as a care provider. Tina had spent a large portion of her pregnancy feeling anxious about the birth because she was concerned about her medical disorder. She had researched her condition along with her pregnancy and knew the associated risks of particular interventions. Her 'research' may have been particular in its focus on her specific health condition, but as I will show, other women in the study who did not suffer from any particular condition were not beyond researching, reading and worrying too.

Grace was a VBAC client of the Cape Town midwives and was excited about the prospect of birthing her singleton baby vaginally.[4] I met with Grace each week from thirty-seven weeks onwards, to the point that she joked that I knew her state and how and whether things were changing even better than the midwives, particularly given that, because of schedule changes, she saw a different midwife each week. When we met a few weeks after the birth, she spoke about the birthing experience. Such conversations were always intense as women described their physical and emotional state during birth. Given that the events were still close in time and that they were adjusting to the demands of new life, including its demands on emotions, bodies and sleep, the accounts were vivid. She described having been anxious to go into labour. She had read about induction and had been anxious to avoid one for fear it would lead to more 'unwanted intervention'.[5] After several 'stretch and sweep' interventions, in which a medical professional runs a finger along the cervix to try and release birth hormones and soften the cervix, and lots of walking, she finally went into labour in the early hours of the morning, the weekend before she was scheduled for an induction. Having been anxious for her natural birth and focusing on that, Grace spoke about the risk she had been unaware of during labour as a VBAC candidate.

> Knowing the risk of rupturing with a VBAC is huge and people asked me did I worry about rupturing. I said, it honestly never crossed my mind, I knew the midwives would never put me at risk and I just knew they had my back and I knew they would never put me in a position of being at risk. Look, no one knows what the body is going to do and I could have ruptured but they just had a manner that helped me not be worried and I think that really helps your birth cos if you're worrying about something maybe I wouldn't push as hard but it never crossed my mind, it's amazing.

Grace, like Tina, 'placed her fears in the hands of the midwives', as clients often put it, to the point that she was vaguely aware of the risks, but these did not 'cross her mind' during labour. Grace describes how she was comfortable that she knew her midwives even though she did not know the full range of risks that came with her condition. Grace located knowing in her midwives. It is ironic that she did this – and was happy not knowing – given that many women believed that obstetricians 'hid' information from their patients. 'Hiding' information was what many women believed established power hierarchies between themselves and their doctors. It was also how women were 'tricked' into unnecessary C-sections when doctors 'hid' details of a baby's size or position. Yet there was a perceived lack of hierarchy for women using midwives. In reality a lack of hierarchy is unlikely. Indeed, MacDonald (2007) notes, trust can impede informed choice because midwives can influence clients and trust can produce situations in which information such as VBAC risk go un-noted. The perceived lack of hierarchy, however, established a relation of trust in midwives.

For Grace, knowledge and planning was not about making herself knowledgeable about VBAC births, rather 'knowing' her midwife and trusting her to care appropriately. Choice and risk were placed in relation to one another: Grace chose how to engage with risk by choosing a specific care provider. It also meant researching in certain ways (for example, about induction) and not others (such as the risks of VBACs). It is worth noting that Grace was referred to as a 'VBAC client': yet she is a woman, not a category. It is common for medical professionals to refer to their patients in terms of their condition or diagnosis. Indeed, I spoke of her as such, internalising how she had referred to herself. Patients can be metaphorically turned into their medical status – a VBAC client. Midwives offered a version of care that seeks to normalise birth and in that normalising, their clients were seen as women, not solely in terms of their risk statuses. With the overarching belief that obstetricians saw their patients in terms of their risk statuses, women using midwives sought care in which they could be seen as women and not risk profiles alone. For Grace, knowing her midwife was also about choosing a carer who would treat her and see her in a particular way. Therefore, being a 'VBAC client' and the associated risks did not define Grace or need to be engaged with heavily by her.

What is not revealed or considered, although it probably informed Grace's 'knowing the midwife', is that the midwives in my study all insisted on obstetric back-up, had licenses to practise and to do so in a third tier (specialist) hospital. Women attempting VBACs were primarily cared for by their obstetrician even though midwives offered most of the labour care. Indeed, in many instances, the obstetrician insisted on being present and assisting at the delivery of the baby, although this was not the case with Grace's obstetrician.[6] Women wanting midwife-attended VBACs are only permitted to birth in hospital and the midwives I worked with did not support women wanting home births after caesareans (HBACs), although there are some unregistered practitioners in the City who will assist with such. The midwives with whom I worked often spoke about the safety of attempting VBACs in most cases but they did not emphasise the point (although it was a given) that should problems arise, they were actually in a hospital where emergency surgery was available at short notice. In other words, there were a series of safety structures that the midwives represented and fronted. Women in my study were able to assume safety as a given because of the people and institutions with whom they birthed.

The framing and expectation of choice and responsibility in making safe decisions alongside the rhetoric of 'best birth' places women in positions of wanting a version of birth that remains 'safe'. Midwifery and natural birth, as MacDonald (2007) argues, are reworked to shape women's expectations of birth. Here the midwife can be seen as 'housing' hospital and safety measures; the midwife stands symbolically as the meeting point between natural birth support and risk aversion. Women saw the midwife as a good choice in the frame of a 'natural' birth in part because, although not necessarily explicitly stated, they knew that the midwives had medical back-up. The binary of 'technical/medicalised' and 'natural' birth operated such that the obstetrician and the midwife came to personify and embody particular expectations and experiences of birth; the former representing 'medicalised' birth and the latter 'natural' despite the fact that midwives were backed up by obstetric practitioners.

Thus when Grace and others handed over their concerns about risk to their midwives, they were indeed handing over risk to medical structures. Women attempting VBACs had less 'choice' because of the VBAC safety parameters of needing to birth in hospital and possibly with their obstetrician present. Yet the ways midwives negotiated these parameters and became a 'front' for safety, offering the option of natural birth alongside (some) decision-making, and allowing Grace and others an imagining of control. Therefore, they were offered a 'natural' birth that still fell within their definitions of natural, despite the apparently contradictory medicalised safety structures in place. Women made decisions about how informed they wished to be and how they engaged with risk, in some cases locating knowing and placing emphasis on a carer. Midwives were part of a repertoire of planning, choices and engagement with the depth and breadth of how women came to inform themselves for the kinds of births they hoped for. As a consumer, Grace was able to choose her carer and how much she knew about VBACs via her midwife: she chose a carer who represented safety but did not engage an (obvious) hierarchical relationship. Grace said that her choices to birth in this way made her feel both 'visible' and 'empowered'; as she said of her C-section birth experience, contrasting it with her 'natural' birth:

> Luckily I was first for the day but we're all sitting there, lambs to the slaughter so there were a lot of things about it that I found disempowering and interestingly, what I can say now, throughout my

> whole [first] pregnancy, was more disempowering because you're in the hands of a surgeon who is going to slice you open and take your baby out.
>
> When you know you're going natural, so even if you end up having a Caesar, when you try for natural, your intention is natural and its 'hey little guy, you and I have to do this thing together, I hope you're lying right [a good position for birth]'. You're visualising, you're reading, you're visualising him lying right and [how] he is going to be and how you're going to be throughout your pregnancy, whereas with Caesar, it's like they're going to slice and take you out so I have no part in that actually, just got to lie still.

Grace suggests that even though she handed risk over to her midwife, she still felt involved, empowered and was recognisable as a critical element in giving birth to her son. Her comment reflects a sentiment similar to the argument made by Carol Laderman (1983) whereby technocratic birth metaphorically removes women from childbirth. Comparing American and Merchang birth, Laderman writes: 'American women are delivered by obstetricians, Merchang women give birth'. This argument travels and applies to the South African women with whom I worked. In this model, 'empowerment' is made complex: Grace willingly handed over aspects of concern, knowing and researching but felt visible, present and involved in her midwife-led birth. I use visible here as a concept to refer to how women using midwives felt that they took 'centre stage' in their births rather than being secondary components to the doctors performing surgery in C-section births. Being involved as the person 'to do the work' of birthing a baby made women feel visible. They were enacting the universal feminine and being seen to do such work. Empowerment, for Grace, was bolstered by visibility. Concepts and sensorial recognition are connected. As Kaufmann (2005) notes of patient autonomy in dying patients, as long as the voice expressing a desire to remain alive was strong enough, that wish was respected. By making and being made visible, Grace's sense of empowerment was honoured and she was recognised as critical in her (and her baby's) birth experience even if realistically, no matter what kind of birth, she experienced herself as essential to the birthing process.

The terms 'give birth' and 'deliver', more than differentiating models of birth, offer a semantic account of the consumer behaviours imagined in the term 'deliver'. While women in my study wished to 'give birth', their behaviour and language suggested that they expected a particular kind of service in which their wishes and 'rights' to birth in particular ways were met. They did not see that being 'involved' and having a sense of 'control' was not a 'right' at all but part of a broader set of privileges. The discourse of 'women's rights' overshadowed the fact that such 'rights' were services to be chosen and were certainly not rights available to all women in South Africa. Women wanted to 'give birth' naturally, but birth needed to be delivered to them in ways that shaped midwives' attentions and care and made women visible.

Locating Trust and Risk

Women using a midwife had often researched the use of midwives and the benefits of a vaginal, unmedicated delivery and in their research, they had learned more about the politics of means of birthing in South Africa. The imagined divides between versions of birth meant that reading on one kind of birth often described other versions of birth and their associated risks. All birth has some form of risk but the divide in birth 'choices' had made risk an axis upon which the perception of choice and choosing between birthing 'options' was sometimes based. I offer an example to demonstrate. Marie was planning a home birth; it had taken some time and conversation with her husband to reach a decision on how she would birth. She explained the process to me when we met in her home one day:

> It's so much more comfortable here [at home] and its really funny, cos when we were in Canada I decided in my head I didn't want to give birth in a hospital in SA 'cos [of] the risk of high Caesarean rates and also, just feeling like the doctor and the team at hospital aren't going to support me in my best interests. And so when I first found out [I was pregnant], I told my husband I wanted a home birth and he was just like 'What! No!', and he didn't want to take any risks and I flipped a switch and I was like, 'It's my baby and I know what it feels like', and he was like, 'Okay, let's look into this' and so he also read the book by Ina May and started researching it and talking to Bridget [the midwife]. He was 100% sold on the home birth, and part of it was even just the recognition that either way we were looking at 30 minutes to get to theatre.

Marie's parameters of risk included unnecessary C-sections and her concern that, by placing herself in an environment such as a hospital, she would end up in a position in which a C-section birth would be more likely. Her husband, by contrast, understood risk in terms of the lack of safety measures should labour and birth need assistance. He imagined that being in a hospital environment would quell his fears. The couple negotiated the decision via reading, research, learning and conversation with their midwife Bridget. Marie's last comment on the time it took to get to surgery was in relation to the fact that should a C-section become necessary, the surgeon, anaesthetist and theatre would all need to be readied and so whether she was coming from home or waiting in the labour ward, there would be a similar waiting period. Indeed, further elucidating Marie's comment about her 'best interests', she said:

> I just want someone who is really supportive and cheering me on, [saying] you can do this *naturally*. So literally, the day after I found out I was pregnant, we were back in Canada, I started researching midwives. Here was different though, I spoke to my friends. I mean, don't you even want to know how much time the doctor is going to spend with you, like, can you get up and walk, like you never thought of any of these options.

Marie and her husband understood risk and care in terms of time, environment, options and support. The idea of having support and her own space animated the natural birth model experience. Risk constituted being in a space where one could 'easily' be taken to surgery. Marie's husband had to 're-learn' and re-define risk, engaging a different relationship with ideas of safety and space in order to support Marie as she navigated decisions about birthing processes.

Here, space and notions of safety were inverted and, as MacDonald (2007: 131, drawing on Ong 1995) calls it, 'reterritorialized': ideas of home were rejected and re-defined. Emerging from a broader historical framing of public and private space and their gendered associations, along with the legal arrangements with home space for birthing (in some cases it would not be covered by insurance or considered legal), hospitals have typically been established as the rationally orientated, obstetric-led, safe space for birthing. In attempting to avert lack of control and choice, Marie did not reflect on the feminist associations with home; a space that confined women (MacDonald 2007: 142). For feminists the home has historically been constituted as a site of female oppression, but for Marie, it was a generative site because she felt 'at home' there and could choose who would be with her. For Marie, risk was defined in terms of her pregnancy plans unravelling easily in an unsupportive environment. Marie was constructing risk in terms of surgical birth being riskier than 'natural' birth and apparatuses that would derail her plans. Indeed, for Marie, undoing or losing her choices constituted risk. Planning therefore offsets risk.

Hunt et al. (2006) describe risk as having multiple meanings in prenatal genetic counselling, specifically in the context of patients and medical professionals' interactions, where making a decision often rests on weighing up risks for which patients are untrained. Clinical and lay notions of risk can be complex and contested: as Hunt et al. (2006) show, even though accounts of risk were linguistically similar, there were multiple meanings associated with risk. Finkler (2003) argues that risk calculation can offer 'an illusion of control as well as conceptions of predestination', in the context of genetic inheritance. Marie's 'calculation' emphasised risk in particular environments, and she located safety with midwives who supported her choices, including the choice to birth in what seems (by the logic of medicalised birth) to be the riskier environment of the home.

Indeed, Sobo (1995), Douglas (1992), Lupton (1999) and Nichter (2003) illuminate the anthropological insight of the power relations and matters of control inherent in risk discussions. They show that it is neither a neutral nor objective concept embedded simply in statistics (Hunt et al. 2006). Knowledge and risk go hand in hand; one cannot know all dangers or else one would have to know everything; therefore which kinds of dangers and risks come to matter in different contexts, and how so become important questions to pose (Douglas and Wildavsky 1982). Douglas and Wildavsky (1982: 5) write that 'risk should be seen as a joint product of *knowledge* about the future and *consent* about the most desired prospects'. In other words, there need to be agreements as to what constitutes risk and what gets counted as such. It was precisely to craft such an agreement that Marie and her husband read up on birth and engaged with their midwife.

Formulated differently, Marie and Grace had planned how they would go about their births and with whom. Those plans were made up of agreements that both defined and accounted for risk. Planning and constructions of risk typically account for a 'rational' approach to life and decisions. Indeed, planning disrupts notions of the naturalness of birth. Yet women defined risk in different ways via issues of safety and best birth practices for their baby. Women planned their births in order to attempt the best way possible to ensure the 'right' birth, a standard set by evidence in support of vaginal birth as well as the apparent binary in versions of birth where one birth was 'better' than another (Avishai 2007, Davis-Floyd 1992). As Rayna Rapp (1999) has shown, this model rests on 'living by the numbers', whereby women are both served and controlled by expert knowledge, and in which choice-making was part of being scientifically literate and becoming a 'good mother'. Choosing how to manage one's labouring body as well as one's carers and environments rendered pregnancy and birth as sites to be assessed and managed (Blum 1999). For the women I worked with, planning was part of choice-making, weighing up risk and deciding on a care provider. For them, not having choice – being without a safety net or being in an unconducive environment – produced risk.

Marie remained at the forefront of her birth decisions and space was part of a plan for ensuring she remained heard during her labour. Many women associated hospital with illness and death and argued that pregnancy was not an illness, or the power structures of the doctor-patient relationship were believed to be housed in the hospital space. Marie understood the hospital space as part of the institutionalised disciplinary techniques for producing docile bodies and was clearly concerned about it (Foucault 1977). Grace even differentiated the theatre from the labour room: the former filled with many medical staff, the latter quiet and dark with only her husband and midwife present. Women accounted for spaces differently: theatre, labour rooms and home were negotiated as markers of natural birth according to different sets of parameters. The rhetoric and literature of the good birth, in which a quiet, calm birthing space constituted the good birth, inflected these distinctions. Space was constructed as one of the sites in which choice was either respected or ignored and where natural (good) birth work could happen or not. The overarching safety parameters that dictated where birth would actually happen were made invisible as the midwife fronted safety and offered 'informed choice' when circumstances changed, such as needing to transfer to hospital.

Language, Projects, Control and Risk

The literature on control helps to illuminate Marie's ideas of control and risk. Birth has increasingly come to be framed as a controllable event (Song et al. 2012, Bryant et al. 2007). Offsetting fear and trying to 'achieve' a desired birth process both link to ideas about control, particularly for women who choose surgical birth precisely because it can be controlled (Fenwick et al. 2010, Chadwick and Foster 2013). Yet this was the case for women wanting natural birth too. They offset the 'risks' of surgical and medicalised intervention by planning care that engaged a 'natural' approach to birth and care. Certain kinds of accompanying work and spaces were desired and practiced. Women wanted carers they could trust. In turn, midwives offered attentive care work.

Orit Avishai (2007) has written on how mothering is increasingly shaped by consumerist, technological and professionalised contexts, noting that middle-class women tend to rely on expert advice in their decision-making. Avishai, writing on breastfeeding in North America, suggests that those offering expert advice often establish standards that render women as 'good' or 'bad' mothers depending on whether they meet those standards. Avishai (2007: 136) argues that this leads to the professionalisation of motherhood, as women attempt to meet the standards of 'good' mothering. As women do the work of accounting for the number of ounces of breastmilk their babies consume, the lactating body becomes a managed site and breastfeeding becomes a project that entails research and planning. I found similar ideas among the women in my study. For them, the contrasts in versions of birth and the imaginary of choice, as well as the recent surge in knowledge about the importance of the first 1000 days and vaginal birth for seeding a baby's microbiome and for infant brain development, constructed a South African middle-class version of reproductive work as a project. For the women with whom I worked – clients and midwives alike – the pregnant and labouring body were sites to be managed, and vaginal, natural birth was constituted as not just the 'good' birth but the 'best' birth.

Trust and Choice: Choosing a Carer Who Chooses Choice

The midwife therefore became the meeting point of various forms of information, associated risks and locations for visibility. While Grace represents this as a simple fact, it was not. Midwives were informed by and made decisions in accordance with how women imagined care. For women who had concerns about the general worries of pregnancy and birth, the midwives were tasked with a careful balancing act of keeping women informed, respected and empowered but also not wanting to overload them with 'unnecessary information' that they would experience as burdensome and which might cause them to worry. Midwife Bridget spoke about the difficulties of finding the balance by giving the example of a difficult medical condition, or a baby not yet properly positioned for birth:

> I don't want them to think it's not a problem and then put getting ready for birth off, so it's hard to find a balance. I often have to consciously relax my face. If I'm trying to get baby's heart rate pattern and I'm concentrating but it can look like I'm worried and I have to think, 'just relax your face, put a smile on your face'. You have to be very conscious of what you say and how you say it and your body language, all the time. The thing like baby's position for instance, I want them to improve, if baby is posterior or not well engaged [then] I want them to work on it 'cos it can adversely affect labour but I don't want them to stress, so sometimes it's better to send them a link to read up on the potential problems [online] or else it can also be a huge shock. Giving them time to think about baby being breech before they see the gynae and that they need a Caesar, and then they're on the back foot [if they don't know the potential problems].

I asked Ingrid how she decided what to tell clients in difficult situations and she said:

> I think very carefully about when to start saying things – it would have to be more than 50 /50 'cos I do think fear is very important around birth – and sometimes you're surprised – it all looks like it's going pear-shaped and then its fine. But you also don't want to spring it on them that 'this is a disaster and we're going to theatre in 5 minutes', so I don't want to do that either. So I try and be pretty straightforward with my findings, 'we're not quite on track', so they get a sense of, a gentle way, and I wouldn't use strong language – if it was an emergency I would expect them to comply, but it has to be pretty extreme for that.

In this account, Ingrid is describing a situation in labour in which there might be very little time to make decisions and break news to clients, but her sentiments about being both straight-forward and gentle apply to antenatal care too. For example, Maggie spoke about a client we had seen one morning who had come to the consultation with a rash across her belly and several other symptoms that could have been indicative of a problem later on when it came time to birth:

> Today, with that woman, I could tell her the most gruesome things but she is probably going to google it anyway – I just said, 'Look we need to find out X,Y,Z', and she asked 'what would that mean?'

> I said, 'What it would mean in terms of the pregnancy is that we would manage the first stage of labour very actively cos if it is in fact low platelets it means you can bleed easily' – I gave her information that was concrete enough to go home with. So I didn't want to scare her but I want people to be realistic. I detest the whole airy-fairy, everything is going to be okay talk; I choose my words very carefully and instil a little bit of realism.

Maggie was using pragmatism – despite her commitment to vaginal birth, Maggie was pragmatic in her use of biomedical knowledge and intervention – as a mode for engaging with risk (MacDonald 2007). She supported and promoted natural birth, but that did not stop her from using and acknowledging the place of biomedical interventions. Maggie was weary of women who did not acknowledge risk but knowing about risk was complex: reading on the internet could cause more alarm than was necessary. Maggie knew that many women read extensively about birth and conducted their own research and she tried to find a middle ground between Google searches and the idea that birth did not need to be known about at all as it was an innate ability. Risk was negotiated and defined in different ways in terms of necessary and unnecessary information as well as who communicated risk. Many made use of the internet (see Bessell et al. 2002, Lavender et al. 2003, Lalor et al. 2007, who argue that the internet has value for pregnant women in helping them to feel informed and empowered, but it can also be a source of doubt and worry). Maggie wanted her clients to be prepared for and realistic about birth but she could not control how much they researched or what they would make of the information that they found. Midwives faced challenges when women approached pregnancy as a project, particularly when they 'knew too much'. These challenges included needing to provide women with detailed reasons for why an article on Google, for instance, might have categorised a condition, position of baby or style of birth as risky. Many of these concerns were not shared by the midwives thus in some ways, those kinds of concerns were 'unnecessary' and unlikely according to the midwives' definitions. Women who arrived with many questions and concerns were sometimes described as 'high-maintenance'.

It is important to reflect on what attentive work was happening and being constructed here. The ways in which clinical information was shared was important to the midwives. After all, they had established themselves as the caring alternative to obstetric-led birth which was criticised for scaring women and overriding patient decision-making. Midwives needed to offer a kind of care in which the woman was respected as the primary decision-maker. They wanted women to know when a finding was not positive, and to retain women's trust that they would be respected; how they communicated that knowledge was critical, hence Ingrid and Bridget's emphasis on gentle explanations and relaxed body language. Midwives constantly monitored their tone, words and expressions, particularly when communicating risk, as they tried to ensure that women learned of risks gently. This finding suggests that voice – how women were spoken to – is critical in care work.

Amanda Weidman's (2014) review of work on voice helps to illuminate the ways in which communication is constituted in and as markers for care work. She examines the status of voice in Euro-Western modernity and looks at how anthropology has framed the relationship between voice and identity, subjectivity and publics. Voices are 'material embodiments of social ideology' and can express different qualities (Feld et al. 2004: 332). Timbre, pitch and volume are all part of verbal performance. The ways midwives communicated is therefore critical to interrogating the mode of care being enacted (Lippi-Green 2012). Voice as an analytical focus demonstrates the bodily actions that went into caring in particular ways and draws attention to the relationship between vocal sound and the intended image to be projected (Rahaim 2012). The gentle volume, tone and pitch of communication that characterised midwives' work instantiated the mode of care offered: one of inconspicuous power relations, in turn reflecting a model of natural birth as quiet, gentle and normal. Care work, embodied, material practices of voice and models directing life-giving work were related in constructing a version of care. Voice and communication were critical constituents of the skill of being supportive as midwives. Women were paying for a particular kind of care: a calm, gentle support experience was part of it.

Bridget and Ingrid practised the natural model of birth that emphasised informing women and doing so in ways they believed were supportive. Modes of communication, voice and expression operated as part of the natural birth service package. Women were consumers and how they were cared for was part of a broader framework of choosing a mode of birth and the care providers who would support that choice. Natural birth was seen as innate but there were kinds of care associated with it and midwives offered that care as a service.

Support, Being Supportive and Trust

Support and being supportive are key themes for midwives. As advocates of natural birth, theirs was a supportive rather than a directive role. The midwifery model operated from the premise of informed choice being key and therefore honesty was critical. How that honesty was expressed was integral to the support given. Tone, body language and choice of words merged to produce what midwives called 'gentle' expression. How midwives communicated was for many women understood as their being supportive. This was an important part of the midwifery mode of care: midwives supported natural birth and they supported women. In the framework of birth in South Africa, this is a critical theme. Obstetricians are believed to be unsupportive: they are understood to not give women choice and they do not assist women throughout labour. Therefore, support constituted a large element of how midwifery care was defined. As women felt supported, another relation emerged. Trust was constituted as a combination of support and locating concerns of risk and safety within midwives, as Grace did. Trust was housed in midwives and was actively located in pregnant bodies as women were told to trust their bodies. As Julie Livingston (2012) suggests, trust is neither definite, constant nor inherent in time and space. Patients sometimes have to choose to trust a system, institution or person. Women were told they could trust their bodies but that also meant trusting the person saying those words. Trust is learned and yet is not constant; it vacillates. The careful relations of the midwife as a front for safety systems, their reputations and skill alongside modes of expression came to act as ways of enabling trust. Midwives offered different amounts of information and specific expressions for revealing information in varying circumstances, a skill Bridget expressed as 'finding balance'. Their work came in negotiating and assessing when to say something and when to remain silent while tending to a tenuous relation of trust which could be broken with too much or too little detail, and all of this while trying to ensure that mother and baby were 'doing well'.

Alphonso Lingis (2003: 178) argues that 'what we trust is someone. We trust someone who affirms something though we do not see or cannot understand the evidence or the proof he or she may have'. Lingis' thought is useful for exploring the different relations of trust in care work. Lingis suggests that trust is not constituted by knowing because one can never quite know or predict another person's actions or response. Yet midwives in my study were offering and presenting concrete methods for constructing trust. The language used in relation to trust is important to note. Having to choose to trust offers ways of thinking about this relation in terms of prior-ness and imperative. To trust implies that there is no imperative, that the relation arises from a prior-ness; one 'does' trust. Yet 'choosing' to trust sits oddly against this framing. One can trust without knowing perhaps, but for women in my study, trust appeared to be more than an imperative. There was active planning, researching and thinking that went into choosing a midwife-led birth. Trust was therefore built via the offerings, support and expectations of midwives. Having planned and chosen a midwife however, there was point where women 'had to choose' to trust. Midwives' skill lay in producing trust through two core practices: gentle communication and support. Midwives responded to women's needs with specific skill sets for constructing emotional work. Those skills were key in recognising women's needs. Those needs were directed, made recognisable and supported by plans for care. Women acknowledged their midwives' work and then trusted them. Thus, prior-ness, choice and planning are related to one another in the making of trust. Trust is partly an imperative, and partly constituted by skills. When skills, reputation and support are offered in this context, the imperative to trust is strengthened.

Emotional Work as Care Work

The expectation of particular feelings (and fear of unwanted ones) draws attention to part of the pregnancy as plan that engaged how women felt. Part of the imagined binary of birth models entailed medicalised birth as 'cold' and 'clinical' while the natural birth offered 'warmth', companionship and support for 'women's work'. Women felt they lacked the medical networks and a broader network where how they felt was made important. Marie anticipated the 'endorphin' rush of giving birth, equating the experience to running a marathon. Feeling a certain way and being able to feel at all were part of the repertoire of offerings in midwife-led models of birth. The women I worked with considered both of these to be absent in obstetric-led birth. As MacDonald (2007) suggests, the irony of midwifery is that it offers a rational framework for 'intuition', experiential and emotional knowledge. Women hoped to feel certain emotions and those feelings confirmed the 'rightness' of natural birth: excitement suggested that pregnancy and birth were normal events and feelings of achievement and accomplishment affirmed the 'hard work' and endorphin rush of natural birth.

Women placed emphasis on how they wanted to be treated with regard to information and responses shared and part of their planning included anticipating their care providers' approach. Women hoped for versions of attention and being offered kinds of attention were therefore a desired element of care work. This point asks why attention is perceived as lacking. Rachel's pregnancy story illustrates the anticipation of carers' responses. She and I met three weeks after the birth of her baby boy and we discussed how she had come to use a midwife. Rachel was a Patient Safety Officer and dealt daily with adverse outcomes in medical practice so risk was an important factor for her in choosing a care provider:

> I knew I would really like a midwife birth but I needed someone who has a scientific approach, is very evidence-based, is seriously clued up and is strong enough to manage me because unfortunately my mental model is all about complications, managing complications, managing someone on the brink of death. And the work I do is all about managing adverse events. So when something really bad goes wrong, I wanted to know what their (the midwife's) response to that would be.

Rachel's account of what she wanted differed from Grace's account because she framed it specifically in terms of safety and management and knowing her midwife's skills. Knowing of her midwife's skills had been sufficient for Grace. Interestingly, Rachel saw scientific and evidence-based practice as the means to ensure safety and 'manage' Rachel's personality yet she was very sure of what constituted natural birth and wanted one. Rachel told me that the week before she gave birth she had been doing a fear-release exercise in the hypnobirthing course and that her biggest fear was that she would feel that she had failed should she need a C-section. Indeed, for many women with options for how they birth, a C-section is seen as a failure because women see themselves (and their bodies) as incapable of birthing and believe they have not done universal (and therefore inevitable) feminine work. Despite Rachel's concern over adverse outcomes, her fear was not expressed as the death of herself or her child but about how she birthed. For her, then, as for others with whom I worked, risk was partly constituted as 'failing' in one's plans and choices. This version of imagining risk reflects enormous privilege.

Controlling who was at the birth, their skills and how much one chose to know involved enormous planning, which explains Rachel's fear of failing. If Rachel 'failed' it would mean her plans and project had been ineffective in producing the desired birthing process, although of course ideally it would have been effective in producing the desired birthing outcome – a healthy live baby. The person caring for Rachel and their approach were therefore key factors in Rachel's classification of concerns:

> R: I went to see my doctor, and firstly there was no excitement, no positivity, because I was such an old primigravida. So there I was, in trouble because I shouldn't have left getting pregnant so late. I come to her in excitement. My friends who have just fallen pregnant and their first check-ups, their excitement was that they got to hear the heartbeat. That was my only expectation. I didn't think I'd had a miscarriage so I wanted to hear his or her heartbeat. So I was so excited about that, then I get lectured that I shouldn't have left it so late, so now I was feeling I'm so guilty; 'Oh my goodness, what have I done?' Then obviously my blood pressure is a bit elevated because I'm feeling a bit…
>
> J: Stressed.
>
> R: Yeah, so she says, 'Oh ja, well there is a very good chance you're going to have preeclampsia', and because my mom was diabetic, there's a good chance I'll have gestational diabetes.

Excitement was a core emotion in Rachel's feelings about her first antenatal consultation: she felt it herself, her friends had felt it and she imagined her carer feeling it for her too. Rachel wanted a certain kind of attention (a concept I develop in Chapter 4) that she considered positive and in line with her own feelings. She did not expect to feel guilty leaving the consultation. There were expectations for how Rachel hoped to feel, constituting part of her planning. Being 'lectured' to feel another way – that is, to feel guilty rather than excited – did not accord with Rachel's desire for support. Ironically, the doctor who was concerned about her physical wellbeing was criticised for worrying over safety issues. Rachel wanted a carer who knew how to manage risk, but she did not wish to hear about it. In fact, she wanted a carer who offered specific emotional responses – excitement and support: versions of attention that normalised her pregnancy and birthing plans. Like Grace, midwives represented safety, but that did not mean safety needed to be spoken about.

Rachel Reed (2013) contrasts rites of passage and rites of protection as necessary but conflicting work of midwives. Midwives enact a rite of passage by tending to the boundaries of aloneness and self-trust understood to facilitate a desired birth. Simultaneously though, midwives practice rites of protection: the institutional tasks necessitated by biomedicine and safety. The midwife therefore performs multiple tasks in pregnancy and labour. In line with Reed's thinking on tending to boundaries in labour, the midwives were tending to the boundaries of knowing – both client and institutionally driven. One person cannot know everything. Knowledge and risk are determined by choices that are undergirded by particular social forms that constitute concerns at any given time (Douglas and Wildavsky 1982: 8). The choice of what constitutes risk and knowledge, and the choice of how to live, are made concomitantly. The choice of how to birth and with whom entailed a choice of what to know, what not to know and the kinds of emotions carers should offer.

Knowing, modes of communication and tacit understandings were critical to the kind of attention Rachel hoped for, or even demanded, when she changed from her doctor to her midwife, Bridget. Rachel attempted to create order and plan her experience by defining the emotions she wanted her care provider to offer. The fact that words such as 'failure' animated Rachel's understanding of birth outcomes speaks to the amount of planning women did during pregnancy for birth. Planning engaged an approach to birthing in which modes of achievement and failure marked an outcome. It is clear that Rachel was drawing on a range of feelings in her expectations for care and birth.

Ways of knowing and managing pregnancy incorporated emotional knowing, highlighting the particular kinds of offerings and attention women anticipated as part of their choice-making capacity as consumers and as women engaged in the project of making a good birth and becoming good mothers.

Crafting Reassurance: Learning, Unlearning, Evidence and Comfort

Different sets of emotional work were drawn on and necessitated as women entered the consultation rooms. For example, when I met her at her thirty-week consultation, Melissa, pregnant for the first time, was enjoying her pregnancy. Her partner came to most consultations with her and he liked to ask questions as much as Melissa. During her thirty-week consultation though, Melissa was concerned about her belly size. She said that several people had commented on how 'small' she looked. Maggie, her midwife, frowned and with an abrupt tone (directed at lay people rather than at Melissa) told Melissa that people were inconsiderate and she needed to ignore people and concentrate on the fact that she was growing a healthy baby. Maggie explained that abdominal muscles are different, depending on one's genes, lifestyle and number of pregnancies so it was impossible to say what an average size belly is, especially for lay people.

Maggie relied on biomedical information and expertise to assure Melissa that her belly size was normal. But Melissa's experience was not uncommon. Women frequently worried about their size, as though the site of their bellies was an indicator of the wellbeing of their baby. For example, Mandy was worried that she was 'too big'. Ingrid kept the consultation light-hearted by telling her they would check her measurements and laughing at Mandy's husband's jokes. After measuring her, Ingrid exclaimed 'what a beautiful bump!' and said that all was normal. As an extra confirmation Ingrid spent time feeling the baby to get a sense of its size and explained that the baby felt great too. On a different day when I was monitoring consultations with Ingrid, Mandisa came in. She was thirty-two weeks pregnant. She was concerned that she had diabetes because of glucose in her urine and began crying so Ingrid held her hand and said: 'I understand why you are worried, and that's part of becoming a mum, worrying, but I'm sure it will all be fine, but until they get the results, it's hard not to worry'. Ingrid confirmed that the baby was measuring a little larger than average but the heart rate was perfect and this was 'a happy baby'. Ingrid reassured Mandisa by saying there was medication she could take should the results indicate a problem but until then, everything was healthy so she should try not to worry and she was sure Mandisa would have a normal birth.

Maggie and Ingrid both offered their clients scientific evidence for wellness or reasons for difference: part of their model of natural birth was trying to 'normalise' pregnancy as an essentially healthy experience and they used medical knowledge, their practised skill and empathic communication to do so. They went about comforting Melissa, Mandy and Mandisa in several ways once they had completed an evidence-based check. They held their hands, spoke to the baby and commented in a friendly, warm manner such as 'what a beautiful bump'. Medical, scientific information, coupled with a mode of sensing women's emotional needs and offering comfort, constituted reassurance.

Here I give another example. Leanne was nearing the end of her pregnancy and had gone for a final consultation with her obstetrician to check the size of the baby and that the amniotic fluid levels were normal. She then came to her scheduled meeting with her midwife, Tanya, who chatted to Leanne about the baby's abdominal size that had earlier been assessed by Leanne's obstetrician as 'large'. Leanne was worried about this. Tanya checked the baby's size by feeling the baby with her hands via Tanya's belly and explained that it was normal because she did not have diabetes, adding 'some babies just measure slightly bigger'. Tanya checked with Leanne that she felt the baby was moving frequently and they spoke about the obstetrician telling Leanne not to take omega 3 from thirty-six weeks onwards.[7] Leanne commented on how she struggled to trust her doctor sometimes, feeling that she was being 'scare-mongered', leaving each consultation feeling that 'everything was wrong'. Leanne contrasted this with her experiences at the midwives' consulting rooms, saying she left the midwives feeling that 'everything was right'. Tanya smiled and assured her the pregnancy was 'spot on' but added that doctors are trained for risk and complications so their outlook towards pregnancy could sometimes be different. She cautioned Leanne not to pay too much attention to unnecessary worries.

Leanne's account suggests that she interpreted her different care providers' conversations along the lines of different birth philosophies. Tanya confirmed this. Tanya was attempting to avert Leanne's negative view of her doctor but in so doing, she appeared to affirm the assumed contrasts in birth models that align obstetrics with risk and complications and midwifery with normality. In other words, risk was conflated with 'obstetric talk'. Like Marie, who saw risk as being in a medicalised institution, Leanne was aligning risk with medicalised birth and associated conversations. Leanne was having to engage with questions of how much she needed to know and from whom she wished to learn. Despite the contrast of feeling all was right with her midwife and all was wrong with her obstetrician, Leanne took her doctor's concern seriously, and she was worried. It was not that one account was more accurate than the other, it was about what Leanne wanted to know and how she wanted to feel.

Margaret MacDonald's (2007: 110) account of pragmatism is helpful in explaining Leanne's position. Drawing on Lock and

Kaufert's (1998) idea of pragmatism, in which use of technologies in antenatal care is about more than compliance or resistance, I suggest that women use different technologies (and in Leanne's case, carers) to achieve certain goals, even if they do not 'buy into' the undergirding philosophy. Leanne left her midwives feeling all was 'right' because they used both comforting words offered in gentle tones and expert knowledge to check the baby and thence to produce reassurance. The measurements from the obstetrician together with Tanya's check left Leanne worried but when coupled with Tanya's casual conversation, explanations, solace and warm body language, she was reassured.

It is important to note that the work of reassurance was not only about making women feel a certain way about the information they received.[8] Reassurance was also a method for assisting women to feel a certain way during their pregnancy as a whole. Reassurance was therefore a skill for enacting normalcy of pregnancy. Pregnancy itself and other people's comments about it were largely out of women's control but because they approached birth in terms of having made a choice about the birth and the modes of care associated with it, the process appeared to be controllable. Thus, part of the reassuring work involved midwives' facilitating how women could know and feel. In some ways, reassurance operated as a mode of refusal, fusing comfort and knowledge so that that worry could be set aside or discounted. The idea of pregnancy as plan entailed knowing and managing information and that included unlearning and recognising what women did not want to know.

Ross (2014) notes that the surge in books and information on pregnancy and birth marks the place of education in the making of the good middle-class mother alongside the place of expert knowledge in what used to be characterised as simply 'women's work'. These literatures favour reassurance over surprise by offering standardisations of reproductive events (2014: 52). Yet, as she notes, the result is more often anxiety than reassurance.

Reassurance is about responsiveness. Arthur Kleinman (2009: 4) suggests in his meditation on care work that caregiving is 'empathic imagination, responsibility, witnessing and solidarity'. By offering the skill of support and comfort, the midwives Ingrid and Maggie, whose work I have explored in this chapter, were responsive to their clients' worry. They provided, alongside explanation rooted in 'facts', the human work of empathy in which words and tones of comfort became methods for offsetting concern.

These practices are, for Kleinman (2009), modes of self-cultivation, as people are produced and are made in relation to others. Failures, vacillations and doubt can be recognised as part of responsive emotional work. Relaying information and offering a responsiveness understood as reassurance were skills that required attentiveness to different women. There was a generalisable response to women's anxiety that midwives offered and when women responded, the work of individualised responses was enacted: a hug for some, more explanation for others and a cup of tea for another. There was a toolkit for reassurance: some methods engaged touch, others entailed use of voice and others used practical elements of feeling a baby or measuring a belly. These tools and skills do not accompany books; therefore the connection with a midwife was key.

Sets of expectations, locations and sites of care, safety and emotional work emerged as significant in the ways in which women constructed their imagined birth experiences. An 'empowered experience', along with 'a good birth', would establish women as having enacted the universal feminine work of natural birth as well as making of them 'good mothers': women with the right to choose how they birthed. Accompaniment (via midwives) was anticipated as part of the planning and management of women's pregnancy and birth journeys. Avishai's observation that women approach reproductive work as a project suggests that part of the work of the plan is to make something alien accessible. Emphasis on feelings and emotional work speaks to the critical work of consolation and companionship and raises the question of how women wish to be seen and attended to. The model of natural birth was aligned with emotion, sensing and sentiment. Rachel, Tina, Grace and Marie's desire for this kind of care (apart from wanting a natural birth) raises questions about the place of emotional work, solace and accompaniment in maternal care practices, and suggests that alienation is an important factor to consider in how women imagine birth.

Alienation and Motherhood

Grace and Marie wanted care that gave them voice and visibility. Rachel and women seeking reassurance anticipated specific emotional work from their midwives. As women contrasted models of birth and associated natural birth with attentiveness, an underlying theme of absence is revealed. Why are attention, 'having an experience' and emotional work seen as lacking yet necessary in the work of care and modern maternal care practices?

As Avishai (2007) has noted, reproductive work for the economically elite is made less overwhelming when it is approached as a project: a site that can be managed and controlled. Avishai shows how women used to engaging with life through a goal-orientated approach, coupled with expectations of how to mother by following expert advice, are caught between the difficulties of bodily events and notions of 'how to do it'. The alienating, new, embodied care work of mothering is made less so when it is made into a project. Following Avishai's critique of the literature on breastfeeding as embodied, it is worth commenting on contemporary birth literature.

North American birth literature has largely established a great divide in versions of birth. A prescriptive account for how birth should be emerges in this literature. The critiques of these stark contrasts in birthing models has been offered but what is made clear in my study is that women understood birth in contrasting terms that inflected their experience. Nina, pregnant with her second child, made this clear as she tried to align her feelings on birth with her actual experience:

> J: Will you be more okay with this birth, knowing what's coming?
>
> N: Everybody knows what to do and I know I'll be okay. What I was saying with Dane's birth was, 'millions of women have done this before you, your body is designed to do this. Your body is capable of doing this'.
>
> J: Do you think it's better to know more or less about pregnancy and labour?
>
> N: I was thinking to myself the other day, 'I've already gone through it before with Dane and with him I was in this unknown, and is that a nicer place to be?' Cos no matter how much I researched, I just didn't know and any other stories I heard meant nothing because I didn't have the experience, and now that I have the experience, does that make it easier? And I genuinely can't answer that question cos I'm scared, so there's a part of me that's like, I do know what's coming and I'm scared of that reality, and you are vulnerable, it's pretty scary, the first time, you don't know what's going on, you don't know what your body's doing and now I'm realising the second time, everything is different, every pregnancy is different. But knowing that I've gone through it and its been okay makes it easier so I still can't answer.

Nina struggled to align her experiences with what she learned from her research: in her framing, one simply cannot know birth until one is in it. This is a reasonable understanding, but in light of the hypnobirthing philosophy used by many women, was actually a unique position compared to some of the midwives' other clients. She believed women knew how to birth, invoking an innate feminine ability along with the universality of birth. Having experienced birth however, Nina was caught between an understanding that birth is natural, that she was innately able to birth her son, and her memory of pain and fear and the difficulty of her first birth experience. Nina was struggling to align her ideas of birth and the experience itself because the two ways of knowing did not fit neatly into the conceptualisation of the 'natural' universal model of birth. For Nina, problems arose when her imaginary of birth as natural and controllable did not work. An innate ability to birth did not sit well with pain and difficulty, with not knowing 'how to give birth' or to push, and her fear as her body did things outside her control.

The belief that birth was an embodied, innate ability is offset here by her experience of it as foreign and frightening. Choosing a midwife was part of the birth preparation and begins to address questions of why women wanted emotional work as care. Women were convinced of the naturalness of birth and the importance of the good (vaginal) birth and were invested in the natural birth model. That did not mean, however, that they were able to 'manage' their bodies in the embodied fashion expected. It can be said these women used birth as a technique – a practice like breathing and walking that their bodies 'just did'. The cultural, historical and social inflections of each of these practices was not visible to them; thus, birth was 'natural' (Mauss 1954, Csordas 1994).

A sense of alienation underpinned women's experience. In late capitalism, the body has become a performative self/body and women were performing a version of birth that made them visible as part of what they imagined to be the universal feminine and produced them as good mothers (Featherstone 1991). Yet their bodies and birth did not always go to plan.

Failure was the term expressed in birth not going to plan. Women often saw themselves as either achieving or failing in their births. Failure became the mode by which women predicated and evaluated their experience. Failing leaves one feeling alienated and alone. This reveals why a plan was critical. Failure constituted risk for the women in my study and they went to great lengths to avoid that risk by engaging particular carers, spaces and emotional responses from carers. For example, in the birthing world inhabited by my informants, obstetricians were framed as removing women's choices and sense of empowerment, and Tina, Grace, Marie and Rachel, whose birth experiences and planning have been at the centre of this chapter, went to great lengths to remove themselves from that risk.

In so doing, they constituted themselves as consumers, purchasing a service package that offset risk and attended to the ways they hoped to feel. As previously noted, choice is considered as part of being a modern person and part of the natural birth model. Yet Rhonda Shaw (2002) points out that women engage with flexibility and choice, but when they are unhappy with their birth experience or feel they 'failed' as was the case for women in my study, the 'blame' lies with them for not accounting for risk closely enough or not engaging with 'reflexivity' in determining risk in order to circumvent it. This is part of 'the burden or responsibility of reflexive self-constitution as liberal, rational subjects in the late modern context' (Shaw 2002: 141). As Martin (1997) suggests, the flexible body is only flexible inasmuch as it is part of a framework of particular reproductive bodies.

Framing birth in terms of a 'right' and 'wrong' way alongside senses of achievement and failure point to the defensive modality of middle-class birthing in South Africa. The expected embodied experience of birthing naturally merged with expectations for particular care and emotional responses to escape feelings of alienation as an unattended new mother, unable to align experience with expectations. Visibility and audibility were antidotes to alienation.

The Making of Visible Women and Mothers: Voice and Visibility in Recognition

Nancy Fraser's differentiation of injustices of distribution and injustices of recognition is helpful in exploring the visibility, emotional responses and recognisability women in my study hoped for. Fraser refers to these injustices as forms of harm that inflect social life. She suggests that to be misrecognised is not to be simply devalued or 'looked down on', but to be 'denied the full status of a *full partner* in social interaction and prevented from *participating as a peer* in social life – not as a consequence of a distributive inequity (such as failing to receive one's fair share or resources or "primary goods") but rather as a consequence of *institutionalised* patterns of interpretation and evaluation that constitute one as comparatively unworthy of respect or esteem' (Fraser 1997: 280, emphasis in original). For Fraser, when those patterns are institutionalised, for instance, in medicine, they prevent participation as much as distributive injustices do. Emerging from debates in which economic and material inequality are conflated with misrecognition, Fraser seeks to distinguish the two, showing that injustices of misrecognition are as material as maldistribution. She offers a way of thinking through the institutionalised apparatuses that hold some back, beyond a lacking of resources. In other words, economic harms can be seen as indirect maldistribution and as a consequence of misrecognition. This is important: many political discussions are orientated around the politics of redistribution and multiculturalist debates on recognition (see the critiques offered by Povinelli 2002, Turner 1993, Yuval-Davis 1999, for example). Engaging one and not the other is for Fraser less helpful than seeing the two issues as connected, as social justice requires both redistribution and recognition. Here is a case in which injustices of distribution and recognition were not connected directly but that did not mean recognition of a certain kind was not at stake.

My study is about a group of people for whom liberal democracy works. As liberal subjects, women using independent midwives were economically elite and accessed the privileges of upper-middle-class life and the benefits of being full citizens in political, social and economic terms. These women understand choice to be a right. In fact, it is a privilege. In their choices, and their expectations to be heard and cared for in particular ways, that privilege was being reproduced along racial lines, whereby women able to choose, as a privilege, are not only middle-class, they are largely white.

As these women are benefactors of late liberalism, it is possible to wonder why recognisability and visibility and the construction of risk along these lines have emerged as core themes in care work practiced by independent midwives. Most debates on recognition centre on questions of difference, multiculturalism and minority, and marginalised groups. Indeed, the women with whom I worked took part in a liberal imaginary which 'acts as a social ethics and social technology for distributing the rights and goods, harms and failures of personal and national dreams'. They were among the few in South Africa for whom liberal capitalist democracy works (Povinelli 2002).

Women wanted to be seen and heard, drawing on a rights discourse of empowerment in how they were made visible and heard in the ways they desired. The myth-making process of dichotomised versions of birth, inflected by legal arrangements, moral discourses of good mothering and a politics of birth constituted a voicing of a version of birth that stood for a means of recognising the universal feminine and her right to birth and be empowered. For the women with whom I worked, recognition was about being seen as women and specifically, women embodying the universal feminine. As Elizabeth Povinelli (2002: 134) explains, voicings (social genres) are the past remnants of standardisations of spaces, people and talk that makes communication meaningful in the present. 'Natural birth' is one such voicing and draws on the myths and arrangements that conflate womanhood, the universal feminine, the universal (good) birth and the universal good mother.

The choice-based burden of responsibilities for the self-constituting liberal subject constituted pregnancy as an experience for which an individual was responsible (Shaw 2002). Choice-based responsibility was met by a perceived hierarchical, controlling and disempowering medical establishment, fronted and crystallised at the site of the obstetrician, denying women full status and therefore, full partnership in reproductive work (Fraser 1997). That perception of denial established the parameters upon which women's desire for recognition was based. The universal feminine and its associated discourse of empowerment merged with the liberal, choice-making subject who approached reproduction as a project to be managed and with the consumer who paid for a service (Avishai 2007). Visibility, audibility and the calling forth and expectation of responsive emotional work are core elements in recognition as care work.

Unseen in these women's desires to be visible, acknowledged and cared for in certain ways was the fact that they were able to access the resources that made care as a service both possible and as a consumer-driven practice that they understood as inevitable – a 'right'. I have shown how parameters for risk and safety could change, but having parameters at all is a form of privilege, and so is being seen and heard by one's care provider. Critically, being able to demand a particular kind of care and attention demonstrates a set of privileges that instantiated a version of care by midwives, and also the fact that safety was not factored into direct decision-making because it was inevitable. Privilege, then, is being able to research kinds of birth for being a good mother, rather than worrying about safety – a safe birth is taken as a given. That is enormous privilege. Therefore, the reproduction of privilege in this instance is the ability to prioritise 'choosing' a kind of birth, assuming one will always have a safe one. Certain people in South Africa are able to access and choose a gentle, attentive version of care in which they seek recognition. Those people are largely white and middle-class.

Solace, Responsiveness and Accompaniment in Modern Maternal Care Practices

The burden of responsibility, carrying the weight of 'failing' in bad planning or bad decisions and not adhering or adhering too much to expert advice are part of the construction of the modern mother. Alienation and isolation seem in many ways inevitable. Indeed, as Fiona Ross (2014: 55) describes, the recording of arbitrary facts, such as feeding times and the number of sleeping hours of a new baby, offers some semblance of normality in new motherhood in which there is 'too much time and not enough'.

Midwives had placed themselves as offering alternate care services to obstetric-led birth but they offered more and were asked to give more. Clara Han (2012) notes that care can be understood as a problem: it is an everyday event of tending in small ways to one another. Han's work describes the lives of those living in poverty and precarious life worlds and she explores the messy relations emerging as Chile's state apparatus has transferred care to individuals and families in its failings as a state. The connections and disconnections of everyday life are exposed in the ways in which care is practiced. Han carefully explores how people share and absorb the hardship of others in forms such as 'silent gifts' – for instance, buying a stereo on credit to help 'calm the nerves' of an addicted informal affine.

The worlds of those in Han's Chilean study are vastly different from those inhabited by women in my study. Yet Han's work points to the ways in which people need and choose to attend to one another in silent gestures and delicate forms of accompaniment. For the women in my study, where a sense of alienation was apparent, women came to pay for the kind of care that offered them the gestures, voices and attentions of an affine. As subjects for whom resources could be easily accessed, a strong sense of individuality was revealed in women's choice, control and management of their lives and pregnancy. Yet much anthropological work has provided an insight into the deeply connected ways in which people navigate their life worlds. Angela Garcia's (2010: 112) work on care and heroin users describes how the usual representation of users losing kinship ties is inverted by users building connections with others. Marilyn Strathern (1984) notes that in relations with one another we realise how we are connected and disconnected, always enfolded in relationship. For middle-class women, those relations and connections needed to be purchased. Modern maternal practices were partly constituted by alienation, isolation and the burden of responsibility. The crafting of support, trust and reassurance were vital. The universal feminine to which they aspired was connected to a strong sense of the midwife as a mother/aunt figure (see Chapter 4) and solace and companionship are part of modern maternal care practices. These were critical emotions in recognising women's desires and needs and in responding in ways that made women visible and audible as specific kinds of women. A plan ensured that such work happened. It is ironic, given that women were never actually alone – as they were pregnant – but responsiveness and connection needed to be bought as a service, as ways of balancing the effects of individualistic, capitalistic, liberal approaches to reproductive life and life-giving work.

Notes

1. Understandings of natural birth for those in my study entailed not being in control, a point I explore later.
2. The idea of pregnancy as a plan does not mean these were 'planned pregnancies' in terms of family planning (although most of the pregnancies in my study were planned). Indeed, in South Africa, there is a strong rhetoric of planned pregnancies which, while used differently in this chapter, feeds into ideas of planning and projects that inform South African women's reproductive decision-making.
3. I explore the complexities of this language of 'elective' and 'emergency' in more detail below.
4. I return to how she was referred to as a 'VBAC client' shortly.
5. It is commonly understood by women desiring 'natural' birth that medical intervention leads to more intervention, i.e. an induction can lead to the need for an epidural because of the intensity of labour with induction, which can in turn lead to a C-section.

6. Grace's obstetrician knew the midwives well, having worked with them for a significant period. The obstetrician in this case is also known to be 'relaxed' about VBACs, understanding the risks to be minimal when managed well.
7. there is some debate on whether this thins the blood, which could lead to excessive bleeding at birth.
8. Indeed, 'feeling a certain way' was about normalising pregnancy and vaginal birth. Anxiety and worry often figure the pregnancy experience depending on how risk is framed. The midwives were working to avert such feelings.

Chapter 3

Self-Making

Pain, Language and Metaphor in Birth Stories

In this chapter I use Faye Ginsburg's (1987) notion of procreation stories as a framework for thinking through how women made meaning of their impending births and birth's relation to pain. I put this into conversation with the work of Veena Das. Das (2000) notes that to speak (and vocalise) pain is to call for recognition and acknowledgement. The crafting of rich narratives and pain stories, drawing on everyday cultural tropes, was useful in making impending pain recognisable to others and offered women a clear marker and materialisation of the universal feminine work of natural birth.

I am going to show how the reproduction of race is complex. The women in my study romanticised and imagined a 'rural', 'wild', 'natural', birth, revelling in the idea of 'going primal'. Yet they had the privilege of medical back-up, and specifically, the option of pain relief. The option of pain relief is not inevitable in South Africa. Women birthing in government midwife obstetric units (who are in most cases not white) do not have access to epidurals. Therefore, I describe the ways in which pain in elite offerings of childbirth were romanticised and these ideas of 'natural' birth offered women ways of making meaning from experiencing pain. Yet making meaning from pain in this context existed precisely because women had the choice and option of whether or not to feel it.

Ginsburg (1987), using Bertaux and Kohli's (1984) notion of 'life story', describes procreation stories as 'narratively shaped fragments of more comprehensive life histories'. She looks at how these allowed women to frame and interpret their experiences in an activist abortion debate in which a small town in the US was disrupted by the opening, in 1981, of a women's clinic openly offering abortions (Ginsburg 1987: 624). Ginsburg suggests that procreation stories craft solutions to disruptions in coherent cultural models of reproduction and motherhood. As a story, there are historical, social and personal factors that come to act upon the crafting of those narratives and importantly, life stories offer an account of how 'cultural definitions of the female life course, and social consequences implied, are selected, rejected, reordered and reproduced in new form' (1987: 624). In this chapter, I show how 'the female life course' or becoming a woman was connected to making the self and was reflected in the ways in which women spoke about pain. In opening this discussion, I offer two brief descriptions of women thinking about the relation of pain and birth.

Marie sat in Bridget's consultation room, with her husband, discussing the birth preparation classes available in their neighbourhood as she wanted to 'be prepared for natural birth'. Marie wanted to know what options would be presented if her breech-positioned baby did not change positions. Her pregnancy was only in the second trimester, but Marie was hoping for a 'natural', home-based water birth, unmedicated. Bridget, her midwife, explained that a C-section was often performed when breech babies remained 'feet first' and explained to Marie how an epidural is administered. Marie visibly recoiled at this description: she crossed her legs, folded her arms around herself, frowning. The thought, she explained, of having a needle placed in her spine was worse than any 'natural' pain of childbirth and as Marie later said to me 'I'm really looking forward to experiencing birth'.

Sandy was from Belgium but had settled in Cape Town to do some postgraduate work and was pregnant for the first time. In her first consultation with her midwife Alison she described how she wanted to give birth: in hospital, with no analgesia or any medical intervention in the form of induction or ventouse. (Notice that here, the hospital itself was not equated with medicalised birth.)

The two anecdotes are illustrative of the links women made between pain and natural birth. As in other first consultations, I was surprised by how knowledgeable women were about pregnancy and birth and by the specialised language set used in the form of medical interventions, particularly in relation to pain management. The literature on anthropology and childbirth engages with this relation. Van Hollen (2003) and MacDonald (2007) show how painful childbirth is imbued with meaning. Constructions of gender are implicated within painful birth (van Hollen 2003). By this, van Hollen means that by going through pain, women are understood to gain social capital as women. MacDonald (2007) suggests that having the choice to experience pain reflects empowerment for women. Yet as I have shown, and will address specifically in relation to pain, pain is only empowering inasmuch as it is connected to becoming a particular kind of women and engaging with a particular model of birth. Therefore, pain is not only a physiological experience (see Kleinman and Kleinman 1994). During the year I spent in the midwives' practice, it became common to hear women make strong claims about pain relief, such as the drawbacks to women's recovery and to their baby's well-being and alertness, and how they therefore did not want it. Particular sets of language, metaphor and ideals emerged around pain as themes in midwives' and their clients' conversations, and these were repeated when I interviewed women in their homes. Midwives recommended specific classes to engage with 'coping strategies'; indeed, classes existed to reframe notions of pain. Birthing pain and its management emerged as central in the imaginings of birth held by those with whom I worked.

In this chapter I examine ideas of self-making and ask what is at stake in how women crafted versions of themselves based on how they imagined giving birth. Thus, I pay careful attention to pain, language and metaphor and how these are powerful elements that elucidate the cultural model of 'the good woman', 'the good mother' and 'the good birth'. By looking closely at the language and metaphor used in pain stories, I unpack the metanarrative that links 'natural', 'primal' birth with 'becoming a woman' and being seen as such. I also show how it hinges on an idea of the rural, a significant fact in a country where race inflects social life in multiple ways.

Some women saw pain as a rite of passage in the birth process, or as a gifting process to their baby and others anticipated the physiological endorphin high that came with the extreme condition of giving birth unmedicated. Childbirth classes and books on 'natural' birthing made pain complex: pain was part of the process of birthing but according to the hypnobirthing model of birth (as I will show later), pain is not necessarily part of the birth process, and while discomfort could be expected, it was not 'unmanageable'. Therefore, pain discussions took several paths. I argue that the way in which women spoke about pain reflects moral interpretations of pain and that these were connected to a construction of the self and motherhood. Such choices also became part of a construction of a site in which privilege was reproduced as particular bodies birthed, made meaning and were cared for in specific ways.

Birthing Is Hard Work but Natural: The Midwifery Model of Birth

Catherine, first time pregnant, bubbly and excited to be having a baby, arrived for her booking consultation at sixteen weeks with her husband and a large folder containing all her 'pregnancy admin': ultrasound scans, scan reports and hospital forms. It was at this consultation that she began learning about how she might want to approach the issue of medication and analgesia, having made the decision to be attended to by a midwife. In the booking consultation, Bridget frequently used the analogy of a marathon to speak about birth. Speaking to Catherine, she said: 'Would you be able to just get up and run a marathon? No, well it's the same for birth – you have to train, eat well and get your head and body into the right place; the birth you want doesn't just happen'.

Catherine explained to me when we met in her home a few weeks later that she was not 'big into reading' and laughed as she said she had not read any books on birth but was thinking of doing an antenatal class. Catherine was not 'preparing' much for her birth. Indeed, one cannot actually 'practise' giving birth. Nevertheless, Bridget's comment was opposed to Catherine's philosophy of 'just enjoying the pregnancy'. Bridget's comment cited above is in line with many conversations she had with her clients when they came to see her for a 'chat visit' (a meeting where potential clients were able to discuss how midwives worked and 'get a feel for the midwife' before committing to being in her care) or a booking consultation. When clients asked what they needed to do for the pregnancy and birth, and what they should be reading, Bridget advised them to exercise regularly ('labour is a physical event and you need to be fit'), eat well 'to avoid complications and grow a healthy baby', and she recommended hypnobirthing classes and reading birth literature that encouraged 'natural' birth.

These comments reflect the complexity of birth philosophies: the midwifery model was clearly used by Bridget who tried to show her clients that birth was like other physically taxing events but that did not make it unmanageable. Yet Bridget's model of birth as natural and normal still required preparatory work. The model was premised on empowering women. Here, knowledge was power and preparation produced knowing in ways that normalised birthing, making it appear manageable. Sallie Han (2013) notes in her account of 'ordinary' pregnancy in the United States that even the terms 'ordinary' and 'normal' are socially and culturally inflected. Using the example of the pregnancy test, she argues that this technology has become a standard means of determining if one is pregnant, a certainty. Being informed in certain ways has for pregnant women become 'ordinary', and in the midwifery model, knowing is so normalised that knowing in certain ways is 'natural'. However, as Karen Sue Taussig suggests, using Ian Hacking (1996), the normal is 'an existing average (which can be improved upon and as a figure of perfection to which we may progress)' (2009:10). By instantiating the normalness of pregnancy, midwives offered a way of thinking about how pregnancy and birth should be and this was different to Catherine's approach. 'Normal' pregnancies, encouraged in the midwifery model, anticipated knowing and practicing in specific ways.

Most of the midwives recommended these practices. Like Bridget, Ingrid also spoke with clients about managing pain. In her thirty-two-week consultation, for example, Jess spoke of being anxious about the potential pain of childbirth despite enjoying pregnancy and being excited to 'meet' her baby. Jess seemed anxious and hesitant when Ingrid asked if she was okay, as she looked down and clasped her hands tightly. Jess admitted that she was suddenly anxious about the birth because she did not respond well to pain. Jess explained that when she had been in a car accident she had become 'very aggressive' on the pain medication and she was worried that her reaction to pain and stress in labour would play out similarly to her accident ordeal. Ingrid explained that labour would be a different experience and asked if Jess had anyone to talk with who had experienced 'natural' birth. She also asked how supportive Jess imagined her husband would be while she was in labour. After they discussed Jess's options, Ingrid said: 'Pain is normal and it's a productive pain; it's not a pain that [indicates] something is wrong but a pain that [indicates] something is right and your body is designed to cope with it'. She added, 'It's a very humbling experience, being in labour but you're unlikely to faze any of us, we've seen it all'. Her sentiment was repeated by midwives as part of how they assisted women navigate this experience. In speaking about pain, they prepared women for it and normalised it as a 'natural' part of life. Like Bridget, Ingrid engaged with a mode of understanding birth pain as productive. This is common in midwifery care models. MacDonald (2007: 112) speaks of 'pain with purpose' in Canadian midwifery practices. The birth experience and any pain that accompanied it was naturalised by invoking the universality of birth as well as strong ideas of it being 'right': female bodies were 'designed' to birth. Support and having a 'positive' attitude were linked to managing pain and point to the model of mind over matter used by midwives.[1] Attitude in this context meant mentally and emotionally approaching birth in particular ways: being prepared and informed of births' mechanisms and viewing birth as 'normal' and 'natural' became part of a 'good' birthing attitude.

As I became more attuned to birth language invoked during fieldwork it became clear that when speaking about pain, women made use of sets of cultural tropes – metaphors – to engage with pain and create a manageable experience. The anthropological and philosophical literature on pain suggests that pain typically isolates in that it is unspeakable (Scarry 1985). Yet recent ethnographic work on care draws attention to the social dimensions of pain. Julie Livingston (2012) provides an insight into 'the intensely social nature of pain' in a Botswanan oncology ward where cancer patients use humour and talking about pain to counter it where there is a lack of analgesia. I use this framing of pain – as a social experience – in conjunction with language use to begin exploring the moralistic, self-making components of pain talk.

While midwives saw pain as an ordinary and manageable part of birthing, nevertheless, their attitudes were underpinned by a moralistic mode. Working hard, attitude, 'good' preparation and the 'right' support would constitute a manageable birth. This mode, seen as working toward 'normal' birth, because it is 'natural', also therefore connects 'good' births with 'natural' births. Ordinary, normal birth is therefore inflected with particular moral foundations (Han 2013). Ingrid's attempts to reassure her client inadvertently set up a standard such that should Jess not cope, she and her body were doing something 'wrong'. As a trope, the idea of 'bodies designed to birth' was connected to ideas of the universal feminine and the 'right' pain was conflated with this model. The universal feminine was therefore linked to experiencing pain, hard work, working for one's baby and a 'good/right/positive attitude'. These were all definitions of natural birth in the midwifery model, yet they are closely linked to an ethic that advocates hard work: a protestant work ethic. 'Good mothers' were being connected with ideas of 'good women' who worked hard.

The midwifery model, largely established in relation and opposed to medicalised/technocratic birth, internationally and locally, seeks to 'restore' birth to women in the sense of allowing women to make decisions about their birth experiences and 'trusting' themselves and their bodies. 'Rightness', 'productive' and 'good' pain are clearly linked to ideas of trust and locating it in the body. I expand on this point below.

Medicalised versions of birth were opposed by the midwives (despite the overlaps). They opposed medicalised birth because of the underpinnings that established a version of birth in which women and their bodies were 'inadequate', thus surgical and medical intervention were necessitated (Davis-Floyd 1994). Removing pain was part of medicalised birth but, according to the natural model of birth, in so doing, women's autonomy and right to birth were removed too. It is worth commenting on the discourse used here in birthing talk. The 'right' to birth is an odd statement. Birth is an event that occurs in female bodies outside of rights. The powerful second-wave feminist discourse underpinning birthing models is therefore revealed in the 'right to birth'. Experiencing the pain of childbirth was linked to a broader imaginary that women's bodies had been metaphorically 'taken over' by medicalised birth models. Birthing in pain – enacting the 'right to birth' – is revealed as making a woman a 'good' (feminist) woman.

The midwives' model, seeking to allow women an experience of birth that would be 'empowering' and 'positive', needed to reframe all the elements of birth deemed 'natural'. This reframing needed to happen because a moral imperative underpinned birthing 'naturally': good births happened outside technocratic models of birth but 'good' births could be painful. Thus birth needed to be reframed as natural: 'good' and 'natural' births were conflated. Feeling labour was part of that experience. Therefore, pain needed to be reframed in particular terms: as 'right', 'good' and 'productive'. These terms were connected to notions of truth: the midwifery project was one of restoration, returning women to the 'true' way of birthing. A mode of the good was therefore connected to notions of truth. The midwifery model thus offered women an option for performing 'true femininity'. Self-sacrificing ideas of suffering and pain were conflated with 'the good' and society's expectations of motherhood as a self-sacrificing endeavour were naturalised (Ginsburg 1987).

Relations between Pain and 'Natural' Birth: Defining 'Natural' Birth

I have shown how those being attended by midwives were acquainted with pain management in terms of the midwifery model of care and birth philosophy. Here, I explore how women imagined 'natural' birth and what parameters defined it as such.

As you recall from the previous chapter, Marie was one of the first women I met during my fieldwork; we set up an interview in her home when she was sixteen weeks pregnant but had met earlier on when she had gone to Bridget for her booking consultation, at twelve weeks. Marie was pregnant for the first time and wanted a home birth. She had carefully researched her options for vaginal birth in South Africa while she was in Canada and had chosen Bridget as her midwife. Bridget came highly recommended by other expats in Cape Town because of her experience of working in the UK. Sitting in Marie's home one morning, she and I started talking about how she had become interested in having an unmedicated home birth without surgical intervention, a birth she described as 'natural'. Marie said:

> Ina May is a midwife in the US and she has a book on breastfeeding that I read for a while and when I fell pregnant I read on labour and delivery and she talks a lot about the decisions that people make, and mostly about the attitude [of labouring women] and I really appreciated [her approach]. She was talking about stalled labours and women who start labour at home and then arrive at the facility and it [the labour process] shuts down, the labour is totally reversed. And women, whose cervix was dilated to like 4/5 centimetres and they arrive at the hospital and because of the interaction with the doctor, it closed to like 2, and so, anyway, I was in the middle of reading this and hearing the experiences of people in SA, the whole tone was negative. [They seemed to suggest that] Labour is terrible, painful, not something you need to put yourself through, painful and whatever we can do to numb ourselves [we should do] and [meanwhile] I'm reading this book by Ina May who is saying women go in like this, and they don't embrace the contractions and it just sets them on this negative spiral that makes the labour worse.

Based on her reading, Marie had begun to learn that there was a strong birth movement in which women were encouraged to 'embrace their contractions' along with 'intervention-free' births. As she describes it above, 'attitude' is a significant factor in how one is able to birth. Attitude, understood as the element of mental work, runs alongside the understanding that pain is part of the natural process of birth. Marie said 'people talk about how your body is made to do this, like its uncomfortable sure, but I can't imagine it's going to be like breaking a bone. Your body is made to do this'. She implied that hospitals, obstetricians – who were seen as 'fronts' for medicalised birth – stall the natural process of labour that would otherwise run smoothly. Marie clearly saw her decision to birth 'naturally' as a stance against 'negativity', 'control' and being numbed by doctors 'controlling' her birth. Like the midwives' model, she presents natural birth as 'the good birth', the 'normal' birth.

As shown above, Marie and others in my study drew on and used particular phrases and sets of language as they anticipated birth. The phrase 'embracing one's contractions', while normalised as a phrase, is odd when thought about outside birth. One cannot 'embrace' a contraction. The phrasing therefore suggests a mode of birthing in which women 'surrender', 'let go' and 'give in' to birthing. Thus, women drew on a set of myths around the primal quality of birth alongside a discourse that seeks to place importance in women's experience – an experience that should be encouraged.

Marie's narrative shared elements with other first-time pregnant women's accounts. For example, Sandy was also expecting her first baby. We began talking in her home when she was twenty weeks pregnant. Sandy's understanding of pain was linked to feelings of 'connection'. She saw birth as a natural experience, steadily eroded by technology. Sandy said:

> Hypnobirthing [explanation below] 100% helps and you look at it a different way, develop a totally different perception of it and what I really like about the course is that it kind of, your understanding just clarifies around what causes the tightening, the pain, and how do you overcome it and it's just a nice mix of the biological side, what actually is happening and obviously giving you the right techniques to mentally stay at ease and prepare yeah so its uh, the pain is definitely a factor and there are ways to deal with it.
>
> J: Would you see the pain as rite of passage?
>
> S: Yeah, for me it is, cos yeah, I don't know if that's silly or not, for me, I've seen it as the normal birthing process and just because there's all this technology out there, that can manipulate the birthing process, I still want to go through that natural, the way women have done it for hundreds of thousands of years. And also, in the hypnobirthing, the book that they give you, it talks a little bit about

> the history, it's quite interesting to read that cos back in the day, even hundreds of years before us, it was seen as something to be looked highly upon, and you know, the women had strength and then obviously it was all manipulated so I just yeah, don't want to lose that in our experience as a woman, to be able to experience that, I think it can be something really special so I do almost see it as a rite of passage, if I'm given the choice, if I'm put in a situation where I don't have a choice, I'll still be fine, I'll still see myself as a strong woman. A lot of importance is put onto the birth [by society].

What Sandy factored out of her account of course was that historically, thousands of women did not have antenatal classes. Specifically, hypnobirthing, the breathing and visualisation course to which Sandy refers, was only created in 1989: it was younger than Sandy. Yet, Sandy drew confidence from her antenatal classes, understanding classes as a means of 'restoring' women to what they should 'naturally' know and be able to do. Restoration was one of the building blocks of natural birth: women understood at least part of the work that they expected of their midwives to involve 'restoring' women to their 'natural state' – a state assumed to be the benchmark defining the 'good'. As in the midwifery model, there was a moralistic mode unfolding as birth was constructed as a means of making a particular kind of woman – a good mother. For women with whom I worked, antenatal classes, yoga, blood tests and ultrasounds at thirteen and twenty weeks were not considered 'unnatural' technologies or interventions, whereas surgery and analgesia were. Particular practices ensuring the safety and certainty of foetal wellbeing were clearly naturalised into women's understandings of 'natural birth' while others remained excluded. Women clearly differentiated intervention along lines of which interventions allowed and disallowed the bodily event of labour and birth. Yet safety was important. Foetal wellbeing and a live baby were important in constituting a (good) mother.

These sentiments reflect the broader picture of birth in South Africa's private health sector. Women had choices in how they birthed and therefore the potentially painful experience of unmedicated vaginal birth was not inevitable. The women in my study were constructing a moralistic mode to reproductive life: a powerful rhetoric of rightness could be used to create a reason and necessity to birth in a particular way. In the next section, I show how morality and character became linked to the cultural model of the good mother.

'Too Posh to Push'

Vanessa met with me on a hot afternoon after her school day was over. She was a Waldorf (Steiner) teacher and felt that her teaching philosophy influenced her feelings on birth. Vanessa was expecting her first child and even though she was in the care of the Cape Town Midwives, we met at the hypnobirthing class we both attended. As we spoke about her reasons for wanting a natural birth, the conversation turned to pain and its management.

J: Are you feeling anxious about the birth?

V: I think you get anxious about it and I've always wanted to go natural – I think initially I wanted an epidural and natural cos basically I wanted the baby to come through the birth canal, that was always my first priority, and then you go through this, well for me personally, I went through phases sort of where you're like it's fine, epidural is okay and then you actually do the research, because when you get pregnant you read everything, and then I read about how an epidural can make the baby a bit drowsy and that causes them to not latch properly and the side effects causes, the injection in your back causes back pain and then I just felt like the natural way, *completely,* is the best way. I found I went through phases and then you feel unsure of yourself...

J: What do you think made you feel unsure of yourself?

V: Listening to other people's stories and then also you hear a lot of the, people who work in medicine are quick to offer caesarean and they talk about the pain. But then I did the hypnobirthing [course] and now I feel, I don't have no fear but I feel, I don't even think about it that much. I used to think about it, literally, for the first, before the hypnobirthing class, daily, I would have a thought, sherbet, how's it going to come out of me, it was a big fear for me. With my Waldorf studies, I also feel like it's the child's rite of passage, to go through the birth process, you know what I mean so I think it's also important for the baby, and the mother. For me, I also feel, you're gonna be a mother, you're going to, you should be able to accept the natural process, not take the easy route.

J: Do you think of pain as another rite of passage of sorts?

V: Well, let's call it a challenge, the labour, I think so, there is nothing wrong with a challenge – if something is difficult, it's good for you, it prepares you for something later and it also tests your character, how are you going to cope with it? So I don't think pain, having a difficulty is a bad thing, I think it's good for you, it really shows your character.

Vanessa drew on a model of birth being a rite of passage, not only for herself but for her baby as well. Not wanting her baby to experience the 'drawbacks' of an epidural, she saw birthing as a 'challenge' to be done for her child. Dealing with birth as a challenge, in Vanessa's understanding, reveals one's character. This is an interesting notion because in reality, character does not reflect mothering abilities. How a woman might weather pain does not reflect parenting abilities either. Terms such as 'character', 'challenge', 'being able to cope' and 'being good for you' are important in elucidating what was at stake for women birthing.

It is necessary to look at the model of the good mother, linked to being a good woman and having a good birth, to see what was unfolding in how women spoke about pain and birth. As middle-class women, most of my participants were reading extensively and wished to do 'the best for their baby'. Campaigns on the importance of vaginal, unmedicated birth abound in both natural birthing literature, articles online and those written by birth experts.[2] Emerging from these writings and information is a particular understanding of what constitutes the 'good mother'. Indeed, the 'good mother' makes the best decisions for her baby, putting her baby first, even if that means going through a painful birthing experience. A painful experience may indeed be necessary as experts advise women, because babies born without analgesia in their mother's blood stream are claimed to be more alert and begin breastfeeding sooner. Understandings of the good mother are also defined in the practice of exclusive breastfeeding (see Avishai 2007). Thus, a model of the 'good mother' is formulated around a woman who 'does her best' and 'gives all' to her baby. A mode of self-sacrifice emerges. Here, it is clear why Vanessa connected her mode of birth with her character: giving birth vaginally and unmedicated showed that she was doing her best, caring for her baby.

A very different model to Marie's was used: one of connection and gifting the process of natural birth to her baby, a point made by Vanessa as she described giving birth 'naturally', for her baby. It is clear Vanessa had decided on what constituted the 'best birth', which excluded using analgesia. Vanessa drew on an interpretation of pain that gave meaning to her experience: not taking the 'easy route', testing one's 'character' and gifting one's baby with the 'good birth' all marked birthing unmedicated as a worthwhile experience. The efficacy of second-wave feminism is revealed in such framings of Vanessa's body and her sense of self as a woman and mother. My conversation with Lyndsey, a British expat, illuminates this point further:

> L: I definitely feel like elective caesareans are cheating a bit – I was like 'Don't cheat, you've got to go through it to have your baby'. They're cutting a corner, it's not fair.
>
> J: But then isn't an epidural a bit [like cheating], someone numbing you?
>
> L: I don't know, I think it is, cos it is blimming ... yeah it's full on [labour], and yeah I think if there are things to help the pain great, but I think it does slow down [labour, having an epidural] so there are negatives to it. I'm not against it at all but I think an operation, cos there are so many negative effects for the baby to having a caesarean so that's why I'm quite anti that. So everything is still [natural] that if you have an epidural, I think if you can choose, if you go the natural route, I think well done in this country and if you have an epidural that's fine cos I don't know, I just think, 'too posh to push', you've got to.

Lyndsey uses the word 'cheating' to describe an elective C-section. As with Vanessa, she suggests that 'natural' labour is an event one must go through for one's baby. Lyndsey's comments highlight several important threads in this chapter. 'Cheating' is drawn on as a term for describing how some women approach birth and is connected to ideas of morality, notions of character, questions of responsibility and is perhaps most succinctly summed up in the phrase 'being too posh to push'. By suggesting women who 'choose' a C-section (or indeed do not have a choice) are cheating, it is assumed they are unable to take full responsibility for birthing, taking an 'easier', morally dubious route. Vanessa's idea of how to birth changed when she learned of the effects of analgesia on her baby while Lyndsey describes the hard work of pushing, alongside pain, as methods that make a woman 'deserve her baby'. Becoming a mother for Lyndsey meant doing so 'honestly' – the opposite of 'cheating'. Therefore, one's character, sense of morality and the ability and willingness to take responsibility are all assumed within how one births. Coupled with these sentiments, is a feeling that one might be too 'haughty' or 'affected' to have a 'natural' birth. Here, 'the good women' is invoked as a model used to define women and their styles of birth. The clinical, sanitised settings of hospital and medicalised birth are connected to women who are 'too posh' – suggesting these are women unwilling to birth in a 'primal' fashion, as 'nature intended'. A good woman therefore works hard, is not 'above others' and has a particular moral compass and sense of responsibility. Birthing in a way that 'shows' these qualities evidences the 'good birth'; the 'good birth' makes 'the good mother'. It is apparent then that women ascribed criteria and 'levels' for 'good births'.

'Good Mothers' and an Ethics of 'Right' and 'Wrong'

Meaning-making was connected to character development and therefore, doing 'good' work, crafting the self. An ethics of the self is revealed, one that involves women setting themselves up as right against others who are 'wrong'. Indeed, women imagined they were making a choice but at the same time, they were disparaging about other women who make other choices. Steve Parish (1991: 323) suggests that cultural concepts 'render the mind capable of the moral knowing required for persons to live a moral life', which does not mean, however, that people will actually live in a 'moral' way. Importantly, these concepts provide methods for shaping and giving meaning to people's experiences. Likewise, Kaufman (2005) notes that 'language constructs and promotes meaning'. She suggests that specific words and phrases are used in medical settings to affect the way in which people experience events and to justify action. 'Rite of passage', 'character-building', 'gift' and 'a challenge' are examples of such words in my study. The myth of dichotomised birth and best birth practices for baby are cultural concepts, language and tropes that establish parameters upon which 'good' birthing and mothering are based. The women in my study constructed birthing through/despite pain as character building and as a rite of passage. These concepts and words shaped and gave meaning to their imagined experience. The moralistic dimension and specific use of language can be seen as projects for constructing the self (and mother) that women wanted to become. The alignment between birth and rites of passage discourses (something women spoke of frequently) is therefore not a coincidence. Birthing through pain had become a mode towards the construction and organising of an ethics of the self – an ethics of the 'good mother' or, the 'true mother', also the 'natural' mother. These three terms overlapped one another for those in my study as good mothering was connected with the 'natural' birth and its associated practices.

Metaphors, Language, Pain and Self-Making

The way in which women spoke about pain reflects a relationship between moral interpretation of pain and the constitution of the self as a mother. Here, I describe the three tropes frequently used by women in my study to open a discussion into the relationship between language, pain and social life.

When I interviewed women, invariably the conversation turned to pain; I would ask women why they had chosen a midwife-led birth and quickly, our conversations became about natural birth. I asked for clarification of what they meant by 'natural': not having an epidural was a significant marker. Marie said:

> I exercise a lot, do long races but training for, feels like I'm training for something, for a marathon or something like that and so yeah, there's work you have to do before you can cross the finish line but when you do finish it's like this amazing sense of 'Wow! Look what my body did!' and um, so I feel like I haven't really looked at it as you know, connecting to ... women and sisters around the world, you know, connecting into the mother nature, I just look at it as, I know what it feels like to have that endorphin kick after you've pushed yourself physically and I can only imagine, doing this will be so much more than that – the hormones, physically, mentally knowing I've accomplished this and the hormones I know that come with it, I think that's what I'm excited about. Cos I don't actually, it's funny cos ... maybe I'm completely naïve but I have no fear of pain. I don't even think of the contractions as painful at all but I am so scared of having an injection cos I know, I've had medical procedures before and they're awful. Even though you are numb, you still feel bad afterwards and it's just awful so I have absolutely no concern or fear of what it's going to feel like while I'm in labour... . Maybe I'm completely deluding myself...

Marie understood labour as 'hard work', akin to running a marathon, but nothing more than this. She did not link her understanding of pain to the experience of 'millions of other women' or to medicalised understandings of pain. She did not imagine some mythic 'Mother Nature' or intrinsic feminine essence. Her approach was pragmatic. In a similar account, Caro, whose second birth I attended, was initially concerned about natural birth. She was a physician and had experienced many births which appeared unpleasant to her; the fact that women in state care, where she worked, are not offered analgesia accounted for her initial anxiety.

When Caro became pregnant for the first time, she sought advice from Jill, a family member who is a trained doula.

> So I knew her [the doula] and we set up a meeting and she was just lovely, really positive, empowering. And Mike [her partner] was quite keen to do it drug free and I was like 'Are you crazy, have you seen labour? I've seen women screaming and pulling things, begging you [for analgesia]' so we spoke about this and Jill said, 'You know, I think you've been traumatised by your experiences – the births you've witnessed have been very poorly prepared for labour, very poor support so often times there wasn't a partner present and women are left to labour on their own. Our [state] midwives are not very good at supporting women in labour because they are very busy, there's very few. It's not a very, necessarily supportive "space"'. So Jill said she would lend me some videos that are totally on the other side 'cos I think you've been a bit traumatised'.
>
> And I realised, watching these women [in the video], they aren't screaming. The one, home birth, pretty normal looking, sort of like me, parents there, not my vibe but she just, I could see she went into the zone and I could see she focused – she wasn't begging anyone, she wasn't out of control and Jane [birth instructor] also said, this isn't like surgical pain, 'this is like doing a 1000 push ups, by 999 you're done and your arms are burning', this is hectic but she said you get that respite in between and you need to use it and that also made me think about it differently, it's not this continuous pain that you've got to – it comes and goes, you can rest in between.
>
> J: So a sense of achievement?
>
> C: Huge, the hormones helped, people talk about women needing to have normal labour to feel like they're a woman. And I was sort of like for heaven's sake this is the 21st century do we really, but it's true! I totally under-[estimated], that sense of achievement. He was born, on my chest. Jill helped him do the breast crawl. After, Jill put Ryan on Mike's chest and I got in the bath and Mike said, you are grinning like the Cheshire Cat and I was like, 'I can do anything!', like oh my word, I just had that sense of, I'd just given birth but I got up and walked to the bath – I needed a bit of help, but I was like, wow! It was amazing, it was such a sense of wow.
>
> J: Although a women is still a women without it.
>
> C: Yes, and you feel for women who have had elective caesarean, but some women don't want it. But then there are women who really want vaginal but have to have a Caesar and feel a profound

> sense of disappointment so you don't want to emphasise that too much, so I don't talk about that ever. I don't want women to feel inadequate but my word, I totally underestimated it! I'm not much of an athlete but I guess that's how you feel after a marathon, but I don't see myself as a very physically strong person, from a fitness point of view so I thought well maybe there's more to my body than I give it credit for.

Caro, with the influence of Jill, made a connection between painful, traumatising birth experiences and a lack of support. Preparation and support were constructed as a remedy for pain as well as shifting perceptions of birth. Part of Caro's journey entailed renegotiating a relationship with birth. Seeing 'positive' birth videos and support from her doula and partner countered the effects of seeing women 'begging for pain relief'. It is interesting that attitude, perspective and preparation were utilised in women's crafting of how they would manage pain because one cannot 'practise' labour.

Felicity and her husband spoke about pain while meeting with Ingrid for the first time after deciding to use midwives for Felicity's second birth. They used language that compared birth to training for sporting events to speak about pain and being prepared for birth because she is a professional athlete. Felicity described her first birth as traumatic. In her view, the doctor was unsupportive and kept trying to rush the birth with induction, even though she was not close to forty-two weeks' gestation. The speed and pain of the intensity of induction-induced labour gave Felicity no time to 'get into' the labour. Once she had an epidural she was 'unable to feel properly' resulting in a ventouse-assisted birth. These interventions left Felicity unhappy with the birth and feeling that these particular interventions could have been avoided. Felicity and her husband spoke about how they had to 'rip the baby out in the end' and how there was lots of bleeding and an epidural because the pain 'sky rocketed' after the second induction pessary. It had been 'the perfect pregnancy' and Felicity was upset with the birth. As a professional athlete, Felicity described herself as having a very high pain threshold. On this basis, they questioned the doctor's birth choices and Felicity's response to pain. She and her husband described how the pain she experienced was a result of the speed of the induction's work in bringing on labour, rather than the possible alternative: that childbirth is extremely painful. They did not consider that birth could just be painful, beyond any expectations or analogies to athletic work. Like Marie's understanding of pain in labour as akin to training for a marathon, journeying through challenges and hurdles, if they understood their bodies to be working hard, pain would have a different valence.

History and memory are significant. Kleinman (2009) looks at the relationship between memory, narrative and moral experience. Using case studies from his work as a psychiatrist, Kleinman suggests that memory is constructed through and helps to produce moral lives. He pays close attention to how memories and morality are expressed in narrative. Felicity and Marie produced narratives and metaphors that drew on their pasts and they connected these memories to 'hard work' narratives inflected with moral underpinnings.

Marie used the analogy of a marathon to describe how she imagined childbirth. The practices of training, endurance and finally achievement were equated with labour. These ideas were aligned with the midwifery model in which 'pain with purpose' and 'working out' were compared to birth. Narratives of work and the past were coming together to produce a metaphor of purposeful (commonly experienced) pain. Ochs and Capps (1996: 25) note that narrative provides order in 'otherwise disconnected events, creating continuity between past, present and imagined worlds'. Caro and Marie's accounts illustrate the importance of creating order and control: birthing was an event they attempted to control even if it could not actually be ordered, and preparatory devices and narratives that engaged metaphors of the everyday made birth a possible, fulfilling experience. Patching together narrative devices of everyday 'hard work' in becoming a woman made pain manageable in the specific instance of birthing one's child, an important feature in 'making' a woman.

As Caro spoke about birth as manageable albeit hard work, she also drew on a cultural trope that engaged ideas of her body 'going primal', outside her control. I asked:

> J: Is pain part of the process?
>
> C: The knee jerk response is it would be great to do it without pain, but I think upon reflecting, I think often, times in our lives, where we've grown the most are often through difficulties and pain and testing yourself. I wouldn't want it every day but by the same token, it's a sign things are happening in your body and tells you where you're at. I could tell the second time, how things were changing, where I was which I'd never seen in the State hospitals. The midwives would

> say this women needs to go through to labour ward – and I was like how do you know, but you can hear. That wasn't something I was in control of – the moaning, I'm making a big noise, not very polite and acceptable but I didn't care. I got to the point where I had been interacting, and then I couldn't, I put my head down and couldn't talk. It's how I could tell I was at transition.

Caro drew on a sense of an embodied response to labour in which the body 'took over', making noises and moving in ways outside her usual repertoire. While literatures on embodiment show how the split between mind and body is not enacted in the everyday, in practice, the duality still existed in birth language (Lambek 1998).[3] In other words, the mind/body dualism might be shown in ethnographic examples to be undermined, but people still imagine it as a defining construct, as Caro did. Indeed, the split became part of a narrative in which a primal part of the self was revealed, doing universally feminine work. Becoming a woman was therefore linked to doing universal feminine work and women's work was part of a mode of restoration. This restoration included doing natural work, linking them to women across time and space.

As women had sacrificed themselves by enduring pain in the past, women like Heidi would do so too. This would make a woman. Heidi spoke about the comfort of a history of women birthing:

> I think for me it definitely was, you want to go through the pain, I wanted to experience what 100s of thousands of women have gone through before, and I definitely didn't want an epidural or anything because that just didn't appeal to me and I think the midwives are really good at helping you manage your pain, they really know what to do and at what time to push you and when to kind of put you in the bath or whatever and I think the incredible thing about the pain is that once the baby arrives it just stops and there's this incredible sense of relief and you wouldn't experience that if you hadn't experienced that pain.

A rush of 'relief' or an 'endorphin kick' were placed in relation to experiencing pain. Heidi had created a connection between pain and the joyful experience one would not get with analgesia as well as experiencing an event 'millions of women have experienced and will go through'. Heidi constructed and engaged the narrative of the universal. The conventionality of narrative made the birth experience a shared one. Ochs and Capps (1996: 27) describe the ways in which a narrative point of view is made via a 'community's linguistic repertoires'. A particular register and language set informed a 'natural' birth, the work, according to this narrative, done by millions of women. Berman and Slobin (1995) provide an insight into the production of 'verbalised events'. They suggest that, via a 'filtering principle', people are not presented with real life events to be expressed linguistically; rather, experiences are filtered in terms of choice in perspective and the options of any particular language. This filtering constructs 'verbalised events'. Heidi was part of the production of a narrative in which birth was natural because it was universal; she filtered out the fact that millions of women and babies, alongside those who have survived, have died. Universality was naturalised and a mode of 'rightness' was invoked in an experience understood in terms of collectivity and the production of the self in relation to a collective.

Overlapping but distinct, the third trope used in birth and pain preparations involved thinking through pain in 'competition' driven narratives: pain and getting through pain was conflated with achievement and accomplishment. Ingrid frequently said to clients: 'there is a real sense of achievement, having delivered naturally'. Mariam said:

> So I just feel like that, I know I'm, I have these high expectations and I know intellectually and spiritually what it is I'm going to experience but I also have a physical experience which my body knows, so now I have to be more brave. Cos bravery is facing reality, it's not fantasy.

Women drew on a particular ethos in regard to their birthing: if one worked hard, and pushed through the pain, one was rewarded with a rush of euphoria and a strong sense of accomplishment, of 'bravery', because birthing vaginally was seen as a socially sanctioned achievement. A mode of competition and goal-orientated approaches undergirded birth narratives. Metaphors were organising activity in particular ways: birth came to be approached as a goal-based event drawing on language sets foregrounding achievement (Ochs and Capps 1996).

The Work of Metaphor

It is important to note the overlaps in women's narrations of pain: they were neither consistent nor static. It is clear that Caro drew on all three metaphors at different times and stages during her pregnancies and relaying her stories to me. Her narratives are illustrative of the ways in which people engage with narrations of the self. Ochs and Capps (1996) note that the self as flexible and fragmented is a concept well-articulated in postmodern analyses (see Goffman 1957) Havel 1983). People are not 'the same person' from one day or story to the next and Havel (1983) argues that narrative's purpose includes closing the gaps between selves of the past, present and the anticipated, imagined world. Caro's storylines waxed and waned as a neophyte, or first-time participant in this particular rites of passage, in both pregnancies and after her second delivery. Narratives ordered birth but these were constructed haphazardly over the course of reproductive life.

The metaphors women used as they described and imagined their experiences illustrate the ways in which women connected pain and natural birth with becoming a woman. The relations between pain and womanhood are part of a broader metanarrative: the universal feminine. It is worth noting that in my study, women were connecting the universal feminine with a particular idea of motherhood – 'good' mothering. Notions of self-sacrificing and doing one's best for one's baby feed into the narrative of the good mother. Thus, women, advised by literature and experts on the advantages of vaginal, unmedicated childbirth, understood the need to go through pain to give their babies the 'best' birth possible. Pain, therefore, defined the 'good' birth which made the 'good' mother.

One might characterise their strategies for making sense of the potential of pain in life-giving as technologies of the self (Foucault 1977). The metaphors women used to account for labour and its associated pain are, I argue, strategies which reflect their own ethical self-understanding and constitution. Women had constructed a birth narrative in which birthing needed to be done a certain way: they needed to give birth the 'right', 'natural' way to enact the universal feminine work of the good birth. They justified pain in terms of its positive outcomes – a live child, endowed with the material gifts (a biome) and a new self – a mother constituted in terms of certain facts. This was a means-end argument. In terms of strategies, natural birth was naturalised as a 'simple' technique, such as running a marathon or working toward a goal one wanted to achieve. Indeed, women made it seem 'simple' but it is not actually easy to run a marathon. By 'simple', it appears they were drawing on a recognisable event rather than a necessarily easy one. Making the self in new ways and enduring pain were necessary for making good mothers; metaphors drawing on everyday events and practices were connected to self-making as strategies that made pain appear possible.

Language, Time and the Stages of Pregnancy

In this section, I offer an account of the birth preparation classes women attended during their pregnancies. I look specifically at the language and temporal dimensions engaged as well as the modes underpinning models of birth.

When Bridget advised her clients to attend antenatal classes, she recommended they begin the five-week long courses when they were at twenty-eight to thirty weeks gestation. This was to ensure that the class would be finished at thirty-three to thirty-four weeks, safely before 'term' (the time at which it becomes safe to deliver the baby and the baby is considered ready) at thirty-seven weeks and allowing women enough time to practise the breathing techniques they had learned in the classes.

The 'natural' event of pregnancy and birth was being ordered and structured in terms of biomedical framings of time. Women who were seeking 'natural' births had midwives who defined birth in terms of time, a linear, chronological event. Maher (2008) describes the ways in which midwives in her Melbourne study used temporal narratives to assist labouring women. Midwives supporting 'natural' birth in Maher's study used tenses and time to work through labour using expressions such as 'you've done that part, *next* you're going to breathe until you feel like you want to push'. In my study, Tanya kept telling Grace she needed to keeping going 'just half an hour longer' during her labour. Therefore Maher (2008) unsettles the contrast between natural and medicalised birth in terms of time.

Midwives in my study also used temporal parameters to define safety: length of pregnancy and length of labour. These accounts elucidate the powerful marking of pregnant women in terms of time and instantiates how biomedical temporal language came to inform the narratives of women's pregnancies as stages 'they' had reached; these pregnancies were still framed as 'natural' and opposed to biomedical framings of care. Classes offering ways to assist and encourage 'natural' birth relied heavily on time in terms of when the classes were done, 'practice time' and using counting as a method for breathing. Biomedical framings of time, I argue, is part of the broader technologies of the self that were enacted in birth preparation classes.

Language and Natural Birth Preparation Classes

I sat in the antenatal class during a cold autumn evening during loadshedding (scheduled periods of time where electricity was cut due to a shortage), listening to pain relief methods by candlelight. The room was filled with nine couples and one single woman, three midwifery students and myself, seated in three rows in a semi-circle facing the television and the midwife teaching. Beth, who ran the antenatal classes, had allowed Caroline to come and promote her 'relaxation for birth' class in our fifth session. Caroline came round to each of us and asked us to take a piece of ice out of the bucket she passed around. We were tasked with holding the piece of ice for one minute and were told to focus on the feeling in our hand. It felt unpleasant, painful, particularly as it was cold outside, and after a few seconds, the coldness turned into the deep ache that feels as if it's entering one's bones when holding something freezing. After a minute we disposed of the dripping ice and moved onto some breathing and visualisation exercises. After doing this, we repeated the ice-holding exercise and were asked this time, to use one of the exercises we had been taught that focused our attentions away from our aching hands and towards our breathing. Having gone through the ice process twice we spoke of how distracting ourselves made a difference in how we experienced the pain in our hands. This, said Caroline, was illustrative of how we could approach labour since the receptors that register pain in the body are the same receptors involved in labour (the fact that our fingers were somewhat numbed by the first ice exercise went un-noted). The analogy of the ice exercise suggested that if one were able to use 'distracting' exercises, and feel less pain in our hands, the pain of labour could likewise be worked through.

I was sceptical: none of the expecting women in the class, or me, had given birth. The difference, however, was that I had attended births and knew what labour and birthing women looked and sounded like. While the pain of the ice was unpleasant, it certainly did not render any of us shaking, grunting deep, guttural moans, unable to move and vomiting with pain. On one level, the exercise worked: if one could work through a painful event by breathing and visualising, one should theoretically be able to apply that to any painful situation. The expectant women felt confident as they chatted in the tea break: it seemed possible that childbirth did not need to be as painful as they had been led to believe by popular accounts in media, television and other women's retellings of birth, and it seemed there were techniques that ensured the pain of childbirth would be manageable. Now that women had made the choice to birth 'naturally', because it was an event they needed to 'get through' in making the self and offering their babies a 'good' birth, strategies for pain relief included downplaying pain. Indeed, the language of pain came to inform the ways in which women imagined and spoke about how they would get through birth. In the example below, I show how the word 'pain' was removed from women's repertoires by the hypnobirthing classes they attended.

The Language of Hypnobirthing

I began the hypnobirthing course early on in my fieldwork, in the first weeks of spring; we met in the evenings over five Wednesdays. Having learned of hypnobirthing via the midwives, Tina and Vanessa, whom I met in the classes, came to be two of my informants.

Kate, the teacher, came into the room smiling and quickly welcomed us all to the class. She asked us all to introduce ourselves, and the pregnant women, all with varying sized pregnant bellies, were asked how many weeks pregnant they were and if they were having a boy or a girl; they all knew except Tina. Kate asked us what we imagined when we thought about childbirth and we were given pieces of paper to write down the first five words that came into our heads when thinking about birth and listed these on the board behind Kate; words such as 'blood', 'red', 'pain', 'screaming', 'sweating' and 'contractions' were mentioned.

Language use appeared to be critical in constructing the hypnobirthing method. Words were used to define perceptions of birth and Kate considered these the cause of fear of birth. Words produced the narration of childbirth and as Lakoff and Johnson (1980) note, metaphor is pervasive in thought and action, and as concepts, these direct our everyday worlds, how we perceive and live in the world. The framework underpinning hypnobirthing appeared to use language in critical ways and having discussed our associations with birth, Kate set out to undo these.

Kate explained how Marie Mongan, who started hypnobirthing, had gone through labours that were relatively pain-free and manageable but soon became unpleasant when, birthing in the 1950s, she was given analgesia as standard protocol and 'lost control' of her labours and births. In her subsequent pregnancies she found a doctor to support her and Mongan finally 'got the birth she wanted'. This led her to use her training in hypnosis to develop the hypnobirthing techniques. These, she claims, prepare women for 'intervention-free' and manageable births that could sometimes even be pain-free. For Mongan, and many of the midwives with whom I worked, birthing was about more than having a live baby, it was about making sure women had a 'positive birth experience', where they felt cared for, empowered and were not traumatised. Undergirding the idea of the positive birth experience though is the cultural work of creating a certain kind of woman and a particular kind of mother: good women and mothers. The body, in this model, is made to do particular work in birth and postnatally. A positive birth experience enabled women to do 'good' mothering work from early on – being able to walk and care for their babies in ways that women who have surgical births are not.[4] Mongan claimed that what made birth painful was fear and should fear be vanquished, so too, at least in principle, should pain.

Fear was constructed as the cornerstone of pain: it was prior experience, words and visual renditions of birth that produced fear. For Kate, history was relevant to fear of birth because death was common in historical accounts of birth (indeed, dying in childbirth still happens presently although this was not acknowledged by Kate). Both infection and lack of technology led to higher maternal mortality rates but because hygiene is now known to be an important factor in medicine and interventions are available when necessary, fear, according to hypnobirthing, can be relinquished when pregnant couples educate themselves and shift their perceptions of birth. 'Hollywood renderings' of painful birth were also cited as the cause of women's negative associations with birth as well as how multiple players in the form of media stories and friends recounted 'horror' stories of painful birth and births gone awry. The visual elements of everyday life had apparently tainted women's image of pain, partly constituting their stories. Narrative, for Ochs and Capps (1996), includes drawing and visual accounts. These were regarded as significant in women's perceptions of birth and how they would experience birth themselves.

Kate made allusions to historical accounts of pain and death but she was non-specific and vague in what actually caused death. She also did not recognise that women in South Africa are still at risk during birth, with a high maternal mortality rate, and birth remains an event where healthy outcomes are not inevitable. She did not recognise this largely because the women with whom she worked were not those at risk, having access to medicalised care when necessary. It is interesting then that while 'natural' birth was embedded in the past and modern women needed to be restored to birthing naturally, it was the past that accounted for fear and hence pain. Narratives collapsed upon themselves temporally in this account.

Kate spent the rest of the class teaching us the anatomy of labour and birth, and how, when the body is not in a state of fear, labour can happen productively, efficiently and without extreme pain. She spoke about the medicalised language pregnant women become accustomed to and described how, when those words are heard in labour, they can produce fear and stress: words can stall labour. Knowledge and information (of a particular kind, rendered as 'truth') were part of the linguistic composition informing hypnobirthing. Medical terms such as 'oxytocin' and 'cortisol' were used frequently but were not made part of the medicalised language repertoire to which Kate referred. As such, language was germane to the philosophy of hypnobirthing and as we had written up the words associated with fear and birth, we began to undo those associations.

What knowledge counts and gets counted was at stake in hypnobirthing: the class drew on telling women particular ways they should come to know birth and which cultural storylines could be forgotten (Strathern 1995). A specific mode of associations and disassociations was used in relation to one another: one could not 'just' abandon 'negative' renderings of birth; renderings of birth needed to be replaced. What constituted 'positive' and 'negative' accounts of birth was also apposite. Childbirth for all the women described above was extremely painful, raising questions of what constituted extreme optimism (positive accounts) and realism (negative) in the hypnobirthing construct.

Words became tools: 'contraction' was replaced with 'rush', 'surge' or 'wave', 'pushing' became 'birth breathing', 'delivery' became 'birthing'.[5] 'Pain' was replaced by 'tightening' or 'sensations'. In this model, words as tools were powerful. If words replaced others, bodies could respond differently in labour. Words in hypnobirthing were structuring activity for a future event so a temporal dimension orientated towards the future came to act on storylines of pain. Whether or not releasing fear and replacing words worked, the work of language shifted the storylines women crafted in their pregnancies and, later, retelling of births. Metaphors are concepts and these structure activity (Lakoff and Johnson 1980). Lakoff and Johnson (1980) use the example of argument as war. One does not just talk of arguments as war, one wins or loses. Language here was shaping the birth experience. In the classes, the self was being constructed in 'feminine work' and the course offered restoration: hypnobirthing 'revealed' the 'real' way to birth and the tools to uncover what had been 'lost' to medicalised birth: both natural birth and 'pain-free' birth.

Again, it is noteworthy that biomedical terms were the cause of difficult birth but biomedicine is acknowledged as a reason why women need not fear birth anymore as intervention is available when necessary. It is constructed here as both the cause of fear and of feelings of safety. The point below takes this thought further.

Despite the fact that it tends towards the natural, the course rested heavily on a scientific knowledge of hormones and physiology: breathing was done to reduce stress by increasing oxytocin through deep breathing.[6] In between surges, relaxation breathing was utilised and this entailed focused breathing but not necessarily into the abdomen or by counting. By focusing attention on breathing, two objectives would be met: more oxytocin would be released via relaxed breathing and attention would be on breathing rather than on any discomfort, allowing for distractions and less pain, meaning more oxytocin production, which in turn resulted in less pain: a productive cycle of pain management. Finally, when it came to birthing babies, women were taught how to 'breathe their babies down'. Rather than using the standard Valsalva pushing, Kate suggested that calmly 'breathing one's baby down' and out, in the form of 'J-breathing' (breathing down through the abdomen and then breathing a curl at the pelvis, in the shape of the imaginary J), allowed the cervix and pelvis to be fully opened, avoiding the stress of purple-faced pushing.[7]

Letters and words constructed how women would give birth, using images of a J to shape the process of birthing a baby. The words women used were set up to determine their version of birth and experience. Words became a form of armouring: they protected women from the 'negative' associations between birth and fear and armoured women as they attempted 'natural' birth. The classes were preparing women for a gentle, quiet birth but the tools for engaging with pain relied on a combative mode. Indeed, hypnobirthing worked against biomedicine but not only used it as a safety net but engaged its terms and temporal dimensions.

Levi-Strauss (1963) describes the ways in which language and myth are made up of 'bundles of relations' – meaning is produced in particular words and constituents and their arrangements rather than in their relations. In this model, words such as 'wave', 'surge' and 'rush' were utilised because they held no relationship and relations with the word 'pain'. Language was being used as a method for reframing the imaginings and perceptions of birth. The symbolic work and power of words was amplified in these preparations by attempting to order an uncontrollable event. Hypnobirthing taught women they could shape their birth experience via attitude and by changing their perceptions. More broadly, it suggests that women can take an uncontrollable, unknowable event and make it ordered and controlled. Classes were offering a method for transcendence: both transcendence of pain and of particular versions of the self. Therefore, techniques of the self offered tools for constructing a mode of the self that was controlled and able to birth 'the right way'. The metanarrative of doing good, universally feminine work was made possible with such techniques.

The course offers an insight into ideas of meaning making and makings of the self in birth. The literature on birth has extensively detailed natural models of birth as attempts to empower women. I argue that the natural model of birth and its preparatory classes did more than this: the structuring of pregnancy around time, classes and ideas of preparation were technologies of the self. Women were unable to actually practise giving birth and classes offered practices and techniques – breathing, visualising, analogies and listening to quiet music – that regulated the natural birth experience and what was constructed as ordinary (Han 2013). These techniques offered the tools to become a specific version of the self. Despite attempts to remove the word and idea of pain from women's linguistic repertoires, the extent to which pain was foregrounded in discussions on birth is interesting. As a significant element of an unmedicated vaginal birth, pain was a clear marker of 'natural' birth and indicated self-making work at stake. Classes and cultural tropes reveal how language and metaphor enfold and inflect how self-making is imagined and constituted.

Virtue and Techniques: Self-Making and Good Mothers

Cheryl Mattingly (1998) shows the relations between morality and narrative. She does this by contrasting narrative and clinical reasoning whereby rationality defines medical reasoning. Narrative reasoning emphasises motives as causes, connections between personal motives and social worlds, and how narrative asserts 'the good' in a given circumstance. In other words, decisions are inflected by social and subjective contexts. There are therefore multiple avenues available as explanatory models for people's accounts of health decisions. Paul Farmer (1988) helps to elucidate these findings. Farmer describes a Haitian illness, called *move san* which is contracted by some new mothers. It starts in the blood, sometimes affecting breastmilk, making it unsafe for the baby. Farmer describes the ways in which the explanations of several participants in his study offer different interpretations for the illness. It is interpreted by many of his informants as only affecting pregnant and nursing women who have been abused and this reading acts as 'a warning against abuse to women' (1988: 80). The illness acts as a mode of morality around how new mothers are treated and is therefore 'the making public through illness of the likely private transgression against women' (Zigon 2008: 118). A 'moral barometer' is attached to the illness then and reveals the moral interpretations hidden within narratives of illness. The moral barometer of birthing is reflected in women's accounts of the 'rightness' of birthing unmedicated and what constitutes a 'natural' birth and a good birth. Set up as a choice, where a 'responsibilisation' (see Zigon 2008: 116) to birthing 'well' was constructed (see chapter 3), moral interpretations are revealed in women's accounts of how they should birth. Pain was a central element in those moral underpinnings.

Tropes and metaphors, understood as tools, can be seen as modes for 'working on and re-forming the self' (Laidlaw 1995). The self was enfolded in becoming a good mother. An ethics of a particular version of motherhood is revealed. Zigon (2008), in his account of Heather Paxson's (2004) work on modernity and becoming a good mother, suggests that motherhood has become part of a performance of certain social virtues. Indeed, Cecilia van Hollen's (2003) work on Tamil women in India illustrates how pain is inflected with different, context specific meanings in which pain garners social capital (indeed, in a context where access to pain medication is minimal). Van Hollen shows that Tamil constructions of gender and maternity rest on a particular version of painful birth and argues that this is the reason that so many women in her study chose induction. Pain and experiencing 'full' natural birth therefore marked what Julie Livingston (2012: 144) suggests might be a relationship between pain and social personhood through childbirth. By this, Livingston refers to the ways in which the women in her study approached pain slightly differently to men: pain performances (as a social event) can be gendered in subtle ways. Where women were able to vocalise their pain, many of the men approached pain as an experience to be endured in silence. Interestingly, it was men who contemplated suicide but were prevented from doing so because of nurses 'continually and deeply socialising his [the men's] pain' (2012: 143). Livingston notes that no woman contemplated suicide, perhaps, she suggests because of the effects of orphaning children and the ways women develop a relationship around pain, social personhood and birth. In other words, a woman endures pain and that makes her a good mother, as a woman who sacrifices herself in varying ways.

Motherhood, and the reproductive work that makes mothers, is not virtuous because it engages social norms. Rather, 'it requires certain kinds of ethical sensibilities properly attuned to one's social world, child and self' (Zigon 2008: 103). A mother, as constructed in the model of the universal feminine, is not necessarily a 'good woman' but is 'good at being a woman'. The classes were direct techniques and modes for being a good woman: preparing, making 'good' choices and responsibly readying oneself for birth and early motherhood. Signe Howell (2003) helps to elucidate this point further. She draws on Faubian's (2001) work on the ethics of kinship and refers to *kinning* as the process by which Norwegian adoptive parents undergo subjectivisation to become a particular kind of person. More than adoptive children becoming Norwegian, people are re-created as new kinds of parents. Birthing naturally, through pain, 'paining' if you will, can be seen in the same light. Pain and preparing for pain were clear markers in which the women in my study took on new social positions, reflected too as moral persons, having prepared for and given birth 'well'.

Recognisable Markers of Women's Work: The Good Mother

I have shown that pain is naturalised in the pain stories women and their midwives relayed. In the model to which they ascribed, women give birth, birth is painful, and therefore pain is part of women's work and women's work makes good mothers. The resemblances to Ginsburg's procreation stories are striking. She notes: 'The location of and responsibility for nurturance in relationship to biological reproduction is of critical concern, the salient value and contradiction for women on both sides of the [abortion] debates'.

Life-giving work in the context of South Africa's duality in birth models is claimed in specific ways. As Ginsburg writes, 'taking a side' acts as 'a source of moral authority for female action' (1987: 627). Life-giving work constructed under notions of the 'right' and 'good' raises questions of how birthing models relate to philosophical questions of 'natural' birth and debates on universal women's work and the right to choose. Indeed, I have shown in this chapter how the self is enfolded into motherhood, a self made in birthing 'naturally'. Women in my study therefore enacted work within the framing of the metanarrative of the universal feminine woman who births in ways that make her a good woman. It also engages with questions around medicalised birth that works, for some women, to take away suffering and discomfort and offers women convenience: both models engage particular stances in terms of feminism and femininity. Indeed, Ginsburg (1987: 633) writes: 'Narratives show how these activists require the "other" in order to exist. This is what gives these stories their dialectical quality; in them the two sides are, by definition, in dialogue with each other, and thus must address the position of their opposition in constituting their own identities'. My informants were crafting identities that existed because of the oppositions in birth models and these identities took on a moral valencing. Pain, for the women in my study, became a key benchmark for assessing the kind of birth one had. How one engaged with pain, attitude and preparation all marked how women birthed and therefore the kind of constructing of the self at stake in 'natural' birth. However, one version of 'true femininity' only existed in relation to its other. The medicalised and natural birth models both draw on specific feminist thought, but for women in my study, only 'the natural birth' could be 'true' or else the other would invalidate the 'duty' and 'necessity' of having a natural birth; after all this was a means-end argument. Indeed, many women in my study were shocked that their friends chose a C-section for the convenience and 'comfort' and described those women as 'lazy' or, as Lyndsey suggested, as 'cheating'. Yet the right to choose and use pain relief is one the suffragettes fought for a century ago (see Greenlees 2015).

For my informants, empowerment, 'working against patriarchy' and doing 'character building work' were how they defined feminist work and their femininity. It is necessary to comment on the concept of 'empowerment' here. Empowerment is used by both 'natural' birth advocates and those who encourage women to make use of medications and procedures that minimise the discomfort of birth. Empowerment in the latter sense means distancing oneself from a sense that birthing is 'women's work'. 'Embracing' (and I use this term specifically as part of the feminist discourse it hinges on) birth or distancing oneself from it marks the ways in which empowerment is utilised as part of a feminist discourse for justifying different kinds of birth. In this book I draw attention to the fact that women and care providers feel the need to justify and choose birth at all. The moralistic underpinnings of birth and how birth is used as an example for either the control or liberation of women's bodies are described in the term empowerment. As I have shown, 'character' and one's ability to parent are not connected to how one births, even if that is how women perceive it. In this sense, how one births should not matter and rather than taking a stance on empowerment, it is important to address why women feel the need to be empowered and seen in particular ways when doing life-giving work. I explore these themes in the subsequent chapter.

It may well be significant then that the majority of women in my sample were affiliated with Christianity and their ideas of character-building, hard work reflects a protestant approach to the body. Ginsburg helps elucidate this point about 'pro-lifers', who appear to hold the same view as the 'natural-birthers' in my study:

> For pro-life women, then, their work is a gesture against what they see as the final triumph of self-interest. In their image of the unborn child ripped from the womb, they have symbolised the final penetration and destruction of the last arena of women's domain thought to be exempt from the truncated relations identified with both male sexuality and commercial exchange: reproduction and motherhood. At a time when wombs can be rented and zygotes are commodities, abortion is understood by right-to-lifers as an emblematic symbol for the increasing commercialisation of human dependency. Their perception of their opponents' gender identity as culturally male – sexual pleasure and individual ambition separated from procreation and nurturant social bonds – is set against their own identification of 'true femininity' with the self-sacrificing traits our culture conflates with motherhood. The interpretation of gender that underpins pro-life arguments, however, is based not on a woman's possession of but in her stance toward her reproductive capacities. Nurturance is achieved rather than natural, as illustrated in the procreation stories in which the point of the narrative is to show that pregnancy and motherhood are accepted despite the ambivalent feelings they produce.

Giving birth 'naturally' was an event that could still exist outside patriarchy and 'control'; it was a method for enacting femininity and maternity, going through the self-sacrificing, character-building event of painful childbirth. Birthing 'naturally' was, for the women I worked with, the method to attain 'true femininity' and 'true motherhood'. Different positions offer a vision for being female. The natural birth model is intended to offset the medicalised birth model. Yet the pain stories in my study illustrate Ginsburg's point that life-giving birth work is achieved rather than natural. Indeed, I have shown the amount of work and 'preparation' that went into imagining and managing such events.

For the women in my study, achievement was conflated with the natural. To experience natural birth was an achievement. Disruptions in reproductive life reflect broader social upheavals and Ginsburg notes that with changes in work patterns for women (applicable to women in my study where almost all had a career), marriage and family formation, and huge advances in reproductive technologies, it is unsurprising that the relationship of women to reproduction has changed. For late modern subjects for whom economic and social apparatus are undergirded by the models of individual autonomy and achievement, these modes are echoed in their birth language and pain stories. So is the fact that these women are consumers, expecting a model of care and a particular version of birth. 'Getting through' pain, perseverance and character development demonstrate a modality in which women felt the need to 'achieve' (and purchase) femininity, or a version thereof, as they crafted versions of the self. That achievement needed to be made visible and recognisable and pain became a method for making clear the work of femininity. Yet they also imagine themselves as part of a solidarity of women across centuries and millennia, often framed mythically and/or romantically.

Pain and Isolation

Why does femininity need to be achieved? In many ways unmedicated vaginal birth is no longer inevitable or necessary. For middle-class women for whom choice is the axis upon which they engage with reproductive life, meaning is created in relation to the privilege of choice. That meaning has been conflated with femininity: bringing life forth in a way that is understood as the work 'women were designed to do'. Vaginal birth, with the pain that accompanies this version of birth, is what makes a version of feminine work notable to others. It also provides a clear relation between life-giving work and an ethics of the self, created via strategies and practices that constitute technologies of the self (Foucault 1977). Veena Das (1996) suggests that to utter the phrase 'I am in pain' is to call for recognition, to be acknowledged by another. As I have shown, language was critical to women's attitudes and relationship with pain. Yet the language and utterance of pain was also critical in crafting relations with others and the self. It crafted a woman to be seen by others as having enacted 'true femininity' and done 'good' work in the production of the self and their baby – a baby who had been endowed with the 'best start'. Therefore, a crafting and reproduction of how particular bodies were born was at stake. Babies imbued with 'the best start' were mostly born to white, privileged women (apart from all the non-white women in South Africa who birth vaginally and without analgesia because they have no choice). Reproduction of privilege was at stake, linked to ideas of pain that were optional rather than inevitable.

Women had ideals for birthing but their stories came to produce their experience, which was not necessarily in line with how they birthed (Ochs and Capps 1996). It is perhaps ironic or maybe inevitable that for the majority of the women I saw through their pregnancies and births, how they birthed did not turn out as they imagined, and nor did that matter. For some women, having a C-section was not ideal but after the facts of having a C-section, they re-ordered their story to highlight the part of their labours where they felt some contractions. Other women experienced labour as unpleasant but, like Caro, created a storyline where it was worth doing because it was hard, 'worthwhile' work. In different ways, coherent, positive accounts were produced. Despite the strong views women held on 'how they should birth', once the early days of motherhood subsumed them, birth filtered into the background of sleepless nights, constant nappy changes, perpetual feeding and love.

A crafting of the self was at stake in the pain stories women fashioned and told; the production of another being – their baby – often fell out of focus. But once their babies were born, stories were simplified: women had their babies and that, in their definitions, made them women and mothers. It is clear then that the work of pain stories gave women meaning and a sense of necessity and 'responsibilisation' in how they birthed in light of their having choice, when they still had 'choice'. Time is clearly also significant to pain stories: narratives change over time and matter less and more over the course of reproductive life.

The women in my study reveal in their stories that while they have choice, they are calling to be seen and acknowledged in specific ways and this suggests a sense of invisibility and isolation that inflects modern, middle-class life-giving work and motherhood. Pain and its relation to birthing 'the right' way was therefore critical to my informants' constructions of a particular birth experience. Elaine Scarry's (1985) work on pain describes pain as isolating, unmaking work. For Scarry, there is no return to normal life after the pain of torture. Yet my study reveals the links women made between pain and isolation: pain stories were utilised as methods for moving away from a sense of isolation, to experience versions of visibility, recognisability and a sense of self defined by society as women 'good at being women'. This reflects the complexity of pain stories and their linkages to moral barometers and an ethics of the self. Pain gave birthing in a particular way purpose. It connected women to their babies as 'gifting work' and it enabled women to become part of a unity that is universal feminine work and made them recognisable to others as having performed that work.

Notes

1. I return to the idea of mind over matter in birth at a later stage in the chapter.
2. See http://bhekisisa.org/multimedia/2016-10-23-caesarian-section-or-vaginal-birth-which-is-best-for-you for an example. Retrieved 13 May 2019.
3. Following Michael Lambek's (1998) noting that despite the problems and theoretical critiques of mind/body separations, the world people inhabit and craft can still unfold in dualisms.
4. Women who have C-sections are unable to walk as soon as women who birth vaginally and driving in the first six weeks after a C-section is prohibited.
5. See the Appendix for a complete list of language replacements in hypnobirthing.
6. See the Introduction.
7. 'Valsalva pushing, or a variation of this method includes: taking a deep breath as a contraction begins; holding the breath by closing the glottis; bearing down forcefully for eight to ten seconds (into the bottom); quickly releasing the breath; taking another deep breath and repeating

this sequence until the contraction has ended (Yildirim and Beji 2008). Directed pushing was introduced in an attempt to shorten the duration of the 'second stage of labour' in the belief that this would improve outcomes for women and babies (Bosomworth and Bettany-Saltikov 2006). This type of pushing has been found to have a number of detrimental consequences for women, including alterations to circulation (Tieks et al. 1995), and increased perineal trauma and long-term effects on bladder function and pelvic floor health (Bosomworth and Bettany-Saltikov 2006; Kopas 2014)' (Rachel Reed, Midwife Thinking in www.midwifethinking.com).

Chapter 4

Making Birthing Relations

The Constitution of Attentiveness and Responsiveness

Having discussed an ethics of the self in the previous chapter, I move the conversation from the self-constituting practices of birthing to a discussion on the ethics of self-care. Therefore, I draw out the methods that went into care work. In doing so, it becomes evident that the relations and figures assumed in the role of the midwife, or the 'expert-aunt', which I explain later, are not only available because care was purchased, but also exist because of the attentions and 'experiences' women expected as they did life-giving work. A relationship with one's midwife that allows for familiarity – such as that experienced by one woman who referred to her midwife as being 'like an expert-aunt' – while perhaps laudable, is certainly not a given or inevitable. Rather, it is a form of entitlement. Therefore, in this chapter, I elaborate on the ways in which care was co-constituted as women approached care with expectations. In doing so, I explore and question the premise from which these women approached birth – as something that should be a (positive) experience. The chapter looks closely at birth as an 'experience' in relation to the availability of accessing a specific carer and the ethics of care.

The body of scholarship that has come to be grouped under the rubric of 'the ethics of care' has tended to either romanticise care or place it entirely as needing to be understood as a service (Daly and Lewis 2000). Care has been assumed to be inherent to women

(Ruddick 1980, Held 1993). The ethics of care literature is vast: emerging alongside feminism, care ethics has centred on questions of vocation, service, class, race and gender relations (Tronto 1989, 1993). The ethics of care has been important in developing ways of thinking through care work and taking seriously the work of care providers as professions and professionals. Joan Tronto challenges the idea that care is confined to a private sphere of life, and is thus gendered female. Ethics of care philosophers seek to move care activities and values to the centre of democratic life (Popke 2006: 506). Relations of trust, mutual obligation and responsiveness have emerged, suggesting that caring and care ethics are an orientation more than an activity in political debates.

Tronto (2005) identifies four virtues of care: attentiveness, responsibility, competence and responsiveness. She uses these as tools that distance care from being a practice specific to any particular group. I offer an account of attentiveness and responsiveness as these materialised in the care work that was practiced throughout my study. Tronto (2005) distinguishes attentiveness as the recognition of another's needs for care and responsiveness as the ways people respond to care. I am going to provide an ethnographic account of how particular terms-of-care materialise in language and practice, which enables a broader conversation on how birth relations are expected and made. Within this account I argue that attentiveness and responsiveness are interwoven. The fact that women in my study purchase their care creates a specific orientation to care. As they are 'purchasers', this element illuminates the co-construction of care: intimacy emerged as a co-produced mode of responsiveness. I argue that the care work practiced by the midwives in my study was responding to an ethics of self-care their clients expressed in terms of 'attentions'. Julie Livingston (2012: 96) states that care giving is moral work and it is both personal and social in quality. She argues that care-giving work is a powerful endeavour: when it is done well, the fragile humanness of compassion, touch and listening are embodied yet when done as work to meet official expectations, it can be interpreted as cold, clinical and lacking (Livingston 2012: 97). It is the social quality of care I seek to describe. Here I offer an account of a mode of care inflected by differentiated birth models and philosophies alongside consumer, choice-based framings of care. I pay close attention to the idea of 'an experience' in both the anticipation and reception of care. Care as 'an experience' provides a way of thinking through how care relations are made, a concept I turn my attention to in this chapter.

Setting the Scene for Midwifery Care

'It's so nice and homey', Natalie commented as she walked into the midwives' consultation room for her first (i.e. booking) appointment. She looked at the photographs on the wall of babies the midwives had delivered (as many women did during fieldwork while they waited for their midwife to finish filling out a form or a pregnancy chart) and remarked on how many pictures there were and how 'cute' the babies looked. The midwives filled out forms and added to charts on a desk facing the wall, so that the midwife and her client faced each other, without a desk between them. Maggie used this lack of distance between herself and her clients to place her hand on their arm or leg while talking to them, often sitting so close their legs would be touching.

The practice was in an old house with wooden floors and fireplaces in the waiting room and the consulting room. All that gave away the fact that the building was not someone's home, from the outside, were the medical plaques on the wall at the front door, detailing each midwife's qualifications and institution of training. The toilet was 'en suite' to the consulting room so women often went to collect a urine sample and their midwives carried on talking with them while they went in after women to do the necessary urine tests. In the hallway, there were pictures of newborns, women in labour and family members, such as siblings and grandparents, meeting a baby for the first time.[1]

Alison's office was warm and inviting with pictures of babies. There were plants, a deep red kilim rug, toys for older siblings to play with in a corner of the room and a scrubbed table with her snacks, paperwork and plants on it. Her desk was positioned against the wall so that her clients, sitting on the big sofa, would face her with no desk between them.

Midwives dressed in clothes that were casual but also smart enough that they did not look like they were 'at home'. Ingrid said, 'I'm such a casual dresser so I like to wear a scarf or something in consults so I look a bit smarter!' Bridget told me how she tried to wear a necklace or a scarf so that she looked 'smart-casual' in consultations with her clients. Tanya's old nurse's uniform was on the back of the consulting room door, but it was never worn during the year I spent with the midwives.

The settings of the midwives' practices offer an entry point into thinking about how a particular version of care was constructed and the kinds of care attributes that materialised. An informal quality to their environment and dress, seen in the design and planning of the practices, suggests a particular tone and timbre to how midwives offered care. Using a house with little marking it as a medical practice removes midwives and their practices from the medicalised versions of birth to which they offered an alternate. The settings offered both a negation of hospitalised, formal environments and an affirmation of qualities associated with home: familiarity, 'casualness' and comfort.

Constituting the Criteria That Define Attentiveness

When interviewing women, one of the first questions I would ask was how they came to be using a midwife and then, why they chose a midwife. In response, women described their ideals, desires, experiences and their expectations of midwives. The common themes that emerged were: 'knowing' their midwife, knowing her 'personality' and how she would accompany them in pregnancy and birth. The following accounts elucidate this point. Jeanne, a medical doctor, who had used the team midwives for all three of her births, spoke of the 'emotional care' of the midwives. I met her when her third baby was eight weeks old. Jeanne was friendly as she jokingly 'shooed' her dog away, and we sat in her garden while her new son slept inside, talking about her birth experiences. Jeanne said:

> What's nice about the independent midwives is that you know them a little. I mean you see them and they're with you from quite early on in labour whereas I think, if you have a gynae and they're supportive, you can also have a very good experience but I don't know if they're always there, you know, they're busy – they won't come when you're 4cm, they wait. So in the early stages of labour it's going to depend on the hospital midwives. It's having the people, the team I think.

Jeanne understood 'knowing' her midwives and their continuous presence over the course of labour not just at the end to be important factors that differentiated their care services from others: she enjoyed the temporal dimension of midwife care in which they were present throughout labour and she felt she had a 'sense' of them. It is significant that Jeanne framed birth and the associated care as 'an experience', a point I explore further shortly.

These factors appeared to be shared qualities among other women. Gill, for example, believed that the C-section she had experienced for her first birth had been unnecessary and she had transferred care for her second pregnancy to midwives, choosing Bridget as her care provider. Gill sat on the floor of her lounge with her baby in front of her, playing. I asked Gill about her second birth experience, which she immediately contrasted with her C-section:

> It was so nice, so intimate, it was just lovely, not a room full of strangers that I didn't know, and afterwards [a Caesar] you're just lying there naked and no one is covering you, you know, stuff like that. I could feel that I didn't have anything draped on me – completely naked. You know its stuff like that, I mean I don't know, I can't tell you for sure, the screen was up but that's what I felt.

> I think just the way Bridget is with people, she looks at you when she speaks to you and she is very sympathetic – a lot of people complain to her and she still just listens and she is extremely caring and just... I never felt rushed in my appointments with her – I felt like if I wanted to speak to her about things and it carried on for 2 hours she would be okay with it and even though it never did, it just never felt rushed, never felt there was anything I couldn't tell her or didn't feel comfortable telling her and also just cos I think she makes herself more available when it comes to smsing when you've got questions, not that I ever really messaged her during my pregnancy, not that I ever needed to but I felt like I could, and that she would be so okay helping me and I think that's also what makes a difference. I think a personality also makes a big difference and I think Bridget isn't an extremely outgoing character, she is quite quiet and reserved which is also lovely and having someone around like that helps a lot.

It is striking that Gill described her second birth as intimate. What marked it as such was having no 'strangers' present and 'knowing' her midwife. Her comments reflect how she understands intimacy and its relation to vulnerability. Gill felt metaphorically and literally naked in her C-section birth because not only was she unacquainted with the full medical team, she felt she did not 'know' them. In contrast, she elaborates on feeling that she could disclose information and 'take time', because Bridget had established a rapport where she was 'available' to Gill. This availability was constructed via a mode of 'open communication' in which clients were able to Whatsapp, call or email Bridget whenever they wanted. Bridget made it clear in each booking consultation that her new client should feel free to 'get in touch' should she have any concerns or worries, or 'just need a chat'. There are several emotional responses and relations described here: knowing the midwife meant feeling comfortable enough to talk, to talk feeling unrushed, and having a sense of the midwife's personality and her availability.

Availability as a core theme presents a relation which is outside typical hierarchical patient-medical professional power relations and is thus an element of care women used to define the midwives' modality, even if doctors, in reality, are equally 'available'. Bridget's 'personality' and 'approachability' were therefore key markers of the kinds of care Gill wanted and what she felt had been lacking in her previous birth: she felt she knew Bridget 'as a person' outside of her professional role. This is ironic because in fact Gill only knew Bridget in a professional role. Nevertheless, the sentiment reflects a desire for attention, and a particular kind of attention at that: 'personal' care in which respective personalities were shared and a carer was available 'like a friend'.

The work of attention here builds on notions of the anticipation, expectation and envisaging of a particular experience. If women knew their carer, and knew she offered availability, a 'normal', 'natural', 'intimate' event could be constructed as an experience, and a positive one. Attention offered women ways of turning their births into 'an experience' and is reflected in the common phrase my informants and their midwives expressed in 'having a positive birthing experience'. Birth was an event being understood as an experience, and specific emotional responses were considered necessary.[2]

Others offered similar descriptions of what they desired from care. For example, Marie was planning a home birth in her apartment during the autumn of 2015. We had long conversations over the course of her pregnancy about how she imagined birth and the importance of birthing vaginally, especially as it would help facilitate breastfeeding, something Marie was both passionate and a little anxious about.[3] She described her expectations for how her midwife would care for her and guide her in labour, taking personality factors into account:

> Ultimately I want someone who is going to be more supportive and to let me lead, but strong enough to intervene if I need her to. Not somebody who I feel won't make me go to hospital even if it's compromising my health or the baby... [The] way that Bridget speaks with authority, but [she] also [respects that] it's your body, she'll follow, like your body is taking the lead. She's quite clear on where she stands medically on things.
>
> So I was looking for somebody with that combination of things that's really *supportive* and *cheerful* but also *letting me lead* the process, but

then if I needed her to, in her answers she was very *strong* about some of the questions around like what you do if you have breech presentation and she was like look, I won't deliver it at home and I was like great, I know where you stand and you won't take any risks with me medically, even if it is my preference.

J: It's really important to be able to trust your carer.

M: Yeah exactly it's a combination of having trust in her ability to make sure you and your baby survive but also that they're going to be really supportive and I want almost a counsellor cos it is such a mental thing. I had someone who had a baby and I asked about her experience and she said, 'I didn't get to make any decisions – when I drank something, whether I had food or not – people make every single decision for me and this is the most important moment in my whole life and I didn't have any ability to control any part of it'. I was like that's terrible, awful, if I wanna have a chocolate bar, I'm gonna have one!

Marie's comment on birth being a 'mental thing' (an interesting notion given that babies are born from bodies!) typifies the importance women placed on the emotional qualities of their midwives. Birth, understood as a mental event, a 'character-building' exercise to be overcome for a 'good birth', needed a particular kind of attention: understood as 'emotional', 'personal' attention.

As we have seen in these extracts from interviews and discussions, all three women wanted personal support, and anticipated that they would get this from midwives who knew them 'well enough' to tend to their specific, individual needs. Personality, 'knowing' the midwife and the midwife knowing her client 'well enough' to support her in a 'personal' manner were important. The typical hierarchical relations between carer and patient were collapsed by these women as they sought a relationship that was personal enough to know 'personalities' (Lock 1993). 'Supportive', 'cheerful', 'letting me lead' and 'strong' are qualities Marie classified as necessary in her care provider. Like Jeanne and Gill, Marie wanted a particular kind of attention: one that allowed her to feel in control, where she 'knew' her midwife and a personality that reflected both a 'cheerful' – friendly – and a 'strong' medical professional role. My informants clearly did not want a carer who did not know what she was doing medically, but desired that the medical aspects of birth be offset by a 'friendly', 'intimate' relation in which personalities were shared.

The desire for this attention is part of the broader framework of birthing in South Africa's private sector. Marie commented that she did not wish to 'feel like a patient', a sentiment that hinges on the argument that pregnancy is not an illness. The midwifery model and its practices sought to work against the notion of pregnancy as sickness. Particular relations were clearly being constituted in response to this. It is important to question why a model and mode of care has been constructed to emphasise 'emotional' care over 'bodily' care in which desiring particular forms of attention is at the core. This speaks to the powerful myth-making process upon which natural birth, as a model, was founded. The women in my study understood birth as 'normal', 'natural' and an event that 'made mothers' and women. Environment, people and 'atmosphere' were all constructed as central to how one was able to birth. Midwives therefore needed to fulfil a very particular role: to be the 'personal', 'available' carer who was aware of and able to support the 'normal', emotional, 'mental' aspects of giving birth. For some women, this role may have even felt 'maternal' or aunt-like. Indeed Lynne described her midwife as being 'like an aunt'. Paying attention to medical concerns alongside emotional ones was necessitated; attention was being crafted in a way that the personal (or creating a sense of sharing personally) acted as a method for shaping an 'experience' contrasted with 'medicalised' care.

Jeanne, Gill and Marie's accounts offer descriptions of the constituent parts of the care relations they desired. 'Supportive', 'strong', 'friendly' and 'available' are the criteria according to which women evaluated care. These qualities become criteria for establishing the kinds of experiences, care and births women envisaged and for valuing them once women were in the midwives' care. The safety net of medical back-up, while important, was overshadowed by how the midwife would respond to safety issues in terms of emotional responses and 'being there'. Attention therefore becomes a feature in birthing care. By offering attention, not only do midwives deliver babies safely; they offer an experience.

Pregnancy, Birth and Care as an Experience

What did midwives' clients mean when they anticipated an 'experience' of birth? I begin with some examples.

Evelyn had transferred to the team midwives late in her pregnancy at thirty-two weeks. Her partner, Andrew, attended each consultation with her. They spoke to Beth about why they had chosen to leave obstetric-led care, saying they had felt rushed during obstetric consultations. Evelyn suggested the consultations had felt as though 'if there was no bleeding, then no worries'. They wanted a version of care that took more than just physiological wellbeing into account and, becoming parents for the first time, they wanted a 'more holistic approach' in consultations.

During the consultation, Beth commented that the baby (in utero) had hiccoughs – she could feel the 'jumping' movement of the foetus every few seconds – but that was very common and often babies had it when they were born too and it did not require any 'treatment'; the hiccoughs would leave on their own both in utero and out. Andrew commented that those were exactly the kinds of 'little details' they wanted from 'the antenatal care experience'. In response, Beth said that she thought technology sometimes got in the way in obstetric-led care; Beth felt that the doctors' use of ultrasound made them 'a little distanced from the baby' whereas midwives used a sense of touch on women's bellies in getting to know a woman and baby in a more embodied fashion.

Andrew presents a desire for care that involves what could be called 'nice but unnecessary details' as part of an experience. Beth locates a relation between the personal and the embodied – distance in this framing is established when the baby is measured and assessed with an ultrasound and not hands. Andrew and Beth – as care receiver and care provider – both reflect on the care experience as one offering 'personal touches'. These touches include 'extra information' and embodied ways of assessing and knowing a pregnancy. By contrast, Andrew and Evelyn, like many others with whom I worked, equated obstetric care and technology with impersonal care work.

A relation between 'an experience', 'the natural' and technology unfolded. Reproductive technologies and the relationship between these and cultural representations have been closely interrogated in the anthropological literature (see Ginsburg and Rapp 1995, Franklin 1997, Morgan 2009). Importantly, Ginsburg and Rapp (1995) note that the extraordinary spread of reproductive technologies has led to complex analyses; these technologies have disturbed notions of 'the natural'.[4]

For women seeking 'natural' birth, the technologies used by their obstetricians unsettles their definitions of the natural and are not considered part of a 'natural birth experience' (or at least these events needed to be minimised: women frequently said they liked the midwives not to provide 'unnecessary' ultrasounds). The Doppler and the midwives' hands are seen as non-invasive and 'natural' – perhaps because the representation with a Doppler is not visual. Therefore Evelyn and Andrew did not experience this mode of representation as invasive. The visual display made possible by ultrasound suggests invasion of a particular kind. There is a sensory distinction between Doppler and ultrasound (the former uses sound waves and even though the latter does so too, there is a visual component). Senses that highlighted sound and touch were clearly preferred by the couple and contributed to their understanding of the midwife offering 'an experience'. An experience becomes a part of 'natural' birthing care, emerging as part of the care anticipated by women and practised by midwives. The wellbeing of a baby could be easily detected via ultrasound (information that these women did not feel lucky to have as they took it as a given) but this failed to provide the embodied 'preparations for parenting' that the slow work of feeling a baby and detecting a heartbeat entailed. The distinction was amplified by Andrew and Beth and came to inform what makes 'an experience'.

That experience entailed slow work and a temporal dimension is therefore connected to notions of embodied care. Hands feeling for wellness excluded certain technologies while including others. This mode therefore aligned with 'the natural' in the birthing myth and the experiences it promised (although almost all the women still used technology for thirteen- and twenty-week Downs' Syndrome and physical wellness scans). There is a model of foetal privacy embedded in these ideas. The womb is imagined as a private space, a bedroom, of sorts. Therefore, using different sensory tools for assessing foetal wellbeing presents an interesting private/public distinction. As the ultrasound is seen as impersonal and invasive, the Doppler and hands feeling a belly 'protect' privacy. Ideas of a baby being 'invaded' suggests particular framings of personhood attributed to the baby and how it is assessed. Midwifery care was presented as 'non-invasive' and 'respectful' of both women and babies. This dimension contributes to the 'experience' of care that midwives were believed to offer.

The bodily knowledge of the midwives as well as their embodied ways of knowing foetal wellbeing linked their knowledge and care to the body and a mode of restoration ('good old-fashioned midwifery'). Bodies that knew how to birth were aligned with expert bodies that knew how to parent and feel wellness in their hands. The senses were connected with the quality of care and how midwives were believed to know about parenting and babies. It is interesting then that women foregrounded emotional care but they appeared to show a preference for an 'embodied' style of knowing. An experience of antenatal care became enfolded into a model of the natural; care became a temporal and bodied relationship. It is important to recognise the emphasis on time and embodiment, which I focus on below.

When Evelyn's pregnancy was thirty-five weeks along, at a consultation with midwife Ingrid, Andrew spoke again about wanting more than just being told 'all was well'. The couple expressed frustration at not having the opportunity to 'just talk' to their former obstetrician. In their view, as far as the doctor was concerned, if there were no problems, there need not be much discussion. Coupled with this, they felt that the doctor 'just went through the motions', using the ultrasound, taking and reading blood pressure. Andrew said 'we want an experience, someone to share in our enjoyment, we want a human, it was so mechanical before'. His comment on 'mechanical' care refers to Andrew's interpretation of how the doctor checked Evelyn and the baby. The assessment was rushed and 'technical'.

The comment arose after Andrew was asked if he wanted to feel the baby (by which the midwife meant that he could place his hands on Evelyn's belly and the midwife would show him where to 'feel' the shoulders, for instance, through the boundary of Evelyn's belly). This was a question midwives regularly asked partners or accompanying parents and children. Andrew was visibly excited as he felt his baby, smiling as Ingrid put her hands on his to guide him to the baby's head and bottom. Andrew said 'I feel so empowered!' and Ingrid, smiling at his comment, asked if he wanted to use the Doppler to hear the baby's heartbeat, which he readily did, although Ingrid had to guide him to the right spot, feeling Evelyn's belly to locate the baby's shoulder to get a clear reading.

Andrew's comment suggests that 'mechanical', 'going through the motions' care work excluded him. Getting to feel his unborn child left him feeling 'empowered', an interesting notion, given that this comment is usually expressed by women in my study, and women in general. Feeling 'empowered', however, was a feeling that Andrew conflated with being involved in the consultation. Beth reflected on her work saying: 'Blood Pressure is important but it's also equally important that your heart feels good when you leave [the consultation]. Ultimately, we want a healthy baby and mom – but it's not just about survival – mom and baby need to feel respected and have a good experience, not just survive'. A 'good' experience, feeling 'respected' and 'empowered' were at the core of the kind of care work midwives understood themselves to be offering: caring was defined as an experience in which women, those accompanying them and the unborn babies too felt a particular way; and care and caring was about more than safe deliveries and surviving.

Like Marie who wanted to feel a certain level of control, or like Gill and Jeanne who wanted to 'know' their midwife 'personally', Andrew wanted to be involved. Being 'involved' reflects another form of experience solicited in the midwives' practice. It is interesting that this comment came from a male partner. It was common during fieldwork for women to express dissatisfaction at the lack of involvement they had in their births (ironic in that they were indeed all essential) but they did not reflect too often on their partner's involvements. Lydia and Ryan, a couple who had been 'trying' to become pregnant for several years, changed from obstetric-led care because they felt that as a couple they did not get 'enough time' and did not create 'a connection' with their care provider.

It is worth pausing here to reflect on the ways a birthing experience was both desired and defined in particular ways. It is intriguing that a key definition entailed involvement and carers 'spending time' with clients and raises the question of why people expecting babies feel uninvolved in antenatal care, wanting 'more time' and why feeling involved is important. I make use of Iris Young's (1984) reflections on subjectivity and alienation during pregnancy to think about this. Young argues that pregnancy undoes the sense of self and affirms phenomenology by undermining Cartesianism and simultaneously undoing the notion of an experiencing, unified subject (1984: 46). Young (1984: 48) writes:

> The first movements of the foetus produce this sense of the splitting subject; the foetus' movements are wholly mine, completely within me, conditioning my experience and space. Only I have access to these movements from their origin, as it were. For months only I can witness this life within me, and it is only under my direction of where to put their hands that others can feel these movements.

Young's insight helps to reveal the unique experience of being deeply involved in pregnancy in the sense of being able to experience it, while subjectivity, as a unified self, is challenged. Young speaks to the notion of bodily, private knowledge and involvement.

Therefore, she offers an account of another version of alienation pregnant women are exposed to. She argues that alienation is a concept used by some feminists to describe a female experience in a male dominated society (see Foreman 1977, Young 1979, Bartky 1982, Greenspan 1983). Young defines alienation as a process in which a subject's experience is defined or controlled by one who does not share the same assumptions or goals. She argues that obstetric care often alienates women from their antenatal and birthing experience. This happens via a process of assuming pregnancy is an illness and extending this notion, using medical instruments that objectify an internal process, devaluing a women's experience of those processes, rendering a lack of control.

Young's writing crystallises the reflections of the women in my study: concerns over control, normalising pregnancy and emphasising the embodied experience of knowing pregnancy. There is a mode of alienation afoot in how women interpret obstetric, technologically driven care. This form of alienation makes it clear why women and their partners, like Andrew, marked involvement as a key element in the care they hoped for. Andrew perceived their doctor as keeping him uninvolved in Evelyn's pregnancy. Evelyn and Andrew saw their former doctor and the technology he used as connected. Hands were not understood as 'the body's first tool'. Thus the use of particular kinds of technology led the couple to feel disconnected and alienated from their 'experience'. The makings of desired subjectivities were undermined by being uninvolved.[5]

The accuracy of these perceptions is in some ways inconsequential to the fact that these understandings were important in how care was understood, anticipated, constructed and practised. They reveal how the opposing models of birth inflected how care was modulated and practised by midwives. Involving women and partners in ways understood as experientially and bodily-orientated was key. 'Natural birth' can be understood then as a cultural model for orientating care that is presented as being opposed to medicalised birth (MacDonald 2007). Indeed, this is not necessarily an accurate perception; this kind of care could easily be offered by an obstetrician. Therefore, 'natural birth' as a category shapes care and constructs pregnancy and birth as a particular experience. The desire for attention and experience draws attention to how women wanted to be cared for.

'Experience' is therefore a critical component in how care is defined and assessed. It was used a criterion upon which to compare care and birthing models as well as those offering care. This need for care as an experience raises the question of why a physiological event needs to be approached as such. Perhaps this is best thought through in terms of the ideas I raised in the previous chapter. A self-making process was underway as people anticipated the birth of their child and their becoming parents. The care called for and invoked constituted an experience because it was a method for constructing the self – a self that was involved and not alienated. Desiring an experience begged a response: responsiveness therefore became key in the midwives' care work.

Constituting Responsiveness in Care Relations: 'Groundedness'

When I began my fieldwork in the spring of 2014, I was anxious about explaining my research and gaining access to work with the midwives, but when I called each midwife to set up a time to meet, I was immediately put at ease by their warmth and friendliness. Once I began sitting in on consultations, my feelings were the same. Women seemed to immediately relax in the presence of their midwives and they spoke about a wide variety of topics.

Alex had trained as a midwife at a military hospital but felt she had only learned how to 'really' be a midwife when she had moved to private practice and apprenticed with one of the more senior independent midwives. During consultations, Alex spoke quickly, moving between questions and advising women: she was always moving and smiled frequently. Women found her reassuring. For example, Zara came into her consultation with sinus problems. Given that ordinary sinus medications could not be used in pregnancy, Alex tried to advise her on alternatives and sympathised, offering comfort and drawing on her own experience. Zara brought up her concerns around the safety of the home birth she desired, so Alex used her own two home births to describe how home births unfolded and why they were safe. Alex reiterated that the rule with home births was that if she told Zara to get in the car, there would be no fighting or questions asked. Zara seemed reassured by Alex's words, her shoulders lowered and she smiled, particularly when it was apparent that Alex would know when to go to hospital. She seemed especially reassured that the decision would not be a negotiation. Reassurance (which I discussed in Chapter 3) in conjunction with conversation on the 'everyday' and Alex's own life and a 'no-nonsense' safety approach to emergencies were the constituent parts of a particular way of speaking with clients that I was seeing regularly the more I sat in on consultations.

Similarly, I sat in a consultation where Alex spoke to Pia about all the errands they still needed to run before the birth. They spoke as if they had known one another for longer than the pregnancy and as if they were picking up from a recent previous conversation: they needed to book Pia in at Mowbray Maternity Hospital and Pia needed to buy a few items for the baby. Alex went about checking Pia's weight, urine, blood pressure, while checking her file and asked how Pia was doing during these checks. Alex empathised with her client's physical concerns, such as itching skin, saying: 'I've had two babies so I know all the ailments of pregnancy', telling Pia to put some vinegar and salt in her bath. Alex used calming, everyday language as she spoke with her clients, addressing Pia as 'my love' and expressed how her sore back was making her feel old. Pia also 'felt old' in her discomfort at being pregnant and they laughed together.

Midwives commonly made use of 'everyday', 'personal' conversation as they did antenatal checks. Tanya used 'everyday' language to talk about medical terms, calling bacteria in the urine test '*goggas*', an Afrikaans colloquial term for bugs, or telling women she was going to do the 'vampire thing' – 'taking bloods'. Maggie referred to most of her clients as 'my love' or '*my skat*', an Afrikaans term of endearment, after initially greeting them by name. Each midwife in her own way drew on everyday, casual conversation. Language used informally and colloquially was an element of 'groundedness' and using conversation that appeared 'personal' constructed a mode of the ordinary that became part of this quality. The 'personal' talk of the everyday was clearly a feature central to constructing a quality of carers that women responded to.

In the care instantiated by the midwifery model, people talked through concerns they had: physical ailments, questions about maternity leave, stories of infertility and concerns around safety and home birth. As a foundation or base, midwives were able to answer women's questions from both their biomedical knowledge and their experience as mothers and women who had been pregnant themselves. That combination worked to make midwives appear calm and sensible in their approach: they were mostly able to answer questions and did so in a composed, relaxed manner.

A telling event was Bridget's surprise when one of her clients remarked that she had seemed anxious when measuring the baby. Bridget exclaimed, 'I try to hide that in my body language!' They laughed about it afterwards and Bridget said she had not really been concerned about the baby's size but did want it checked at the time, 'just to be safe'. Bridget's use of language and her priorities around safety offer reassurance to her clients. Even without the 'personal touches' of presenting herself as 'calm', feeling safe was an important element to care work and Bridget used particular kinds of language and commented in ways that revealed to her clients that she was concerned with safety. This is illustrative of Marie's comment in which safety was an important factor in choosing a midwife. How safety issues were expressed is indeed also important. Thus, the kinds of language used and how it is communicated constitutes a form of responsiveness women enjoyed.

As midwives drew on years of experience and a biomedical training, there were few questions the midwives had never encountered, something they regularly told women: 'Don't worry, there is little we haven't seen or heard'. Thus, midwives were presenting themselves as care givers who took safety seriously and stated this in their language use, but they did so calmly and wove 'safety talk' into everyday conversation. In combination with safety, 'everyday' talk, comfort and personal experience constituted the 'grounded' quality that clients and I experienced. The midwives rarely came across as flustered because they generally were not: they believed that women should birth vaginally and they had the skills to assist in births that turned awry as well as medical back-up in the form of their own training and doctors to call.

Particular relations were established in the work midwives did while interacting with women; specific qualities and attributes were constituted via those relations: a 'grounded persona'. Relations of care were used in specific ways and combinations to construct a version of accompaniment and comportment, a 'grounded' midwife. Care work was being practised and care givers were presenting themselves in accordance with the model of natural birth and the collective imaginary of how natural birthing care should be.

Part of responding to the needs of women entailed constructing a persona. By persona I refer to ideas linked to Erving Goffman's notion of performance. Goffman (1957) argues that people are constantly involved in different kinds of performances with one another and different 'personas' are presented in different contexts. In the midwifery practices, midwives were clearly using a mode of the 'everyday' in conjunction with particular kinds of language and framings of safety to establish themselves as 'grounded'. This, I argue, was a persona because, as I stated earlier, clients did not actually 'know' their midwives personally. Importantly though, they felt that they did: a persona was presented to clients.

More than a response, care is therefore constituted in multiple ways and entails performative elements. Goffman (1957: 42) describes the enormous difficulty in making a conversation or performance feel casual and work effectively. Performance is fragile work: a minor mishap can make a carefully produced persona appear false (Goffman 1957: 43). Interactions between two people are complex because no person has only one role, and not all roles are necessarily committed to equally, yet all people perform different roles in different contexts. Each of us, according to Goffman, have several roles (Goffman 1957 85). Goffman (1957) argued that all people perform roles when there are others around and it is only when no one is looking that 'expression' of the self happens. This sits in a complex relation to the self-making work that requires another that I have addressed. Indeed, this relation suggests that different selves come to bear on self-making. While Goffman is useful in thinking through roles played, my work shows how selves are enfolded into one another. Goffman is useful in thinking through the multiple selves that may come to bear on the self-making of the 'good mother'. Writing from a functionalist perspective, Talcott Parsons (1964) argued that people have functions for society and those functions are role-played with particular sets of expectations and behaviour placed on different role-players. In that way, people come to infer certain kinds of behaviour from others and expect a particular comportment. While not understood as structured in the same way, the essence of Goffman and Parson's arguments remains useful because it demonstrates the ways in which a professional model of care can be made to appear personal. Thus the personas and roles midwives took on reveal their care relations as a practice. Indeed, a practice of 'groundedness' reveals the role midwives took on as a mode of responsiveness. Groundedness meant that midwives were 'seen' in specific ways and that care 'felt' familiar.

Constituting Responsiveness in Care Relations: 'Familiarity'

Ingrid went about her consultations in similar ways to Alex, although being more reserved, she did not use terms of endearment or share quite so much from her own life. An example drawn from

Nora's first consultation demonstrates this. Nora was a new client but had transferred late (at thirty-six weeks) to the team midwives because she described her obstetrician as not offering her 'the experience' they wanted. She began by telling Ingrid how she had been trying to have a baby for six years, with two miscarriages. She had 'suddenly become pregnant'. Ingrid sympathised with her losses but expressed happiness for Nora's carrying to term finally. Ingrid did her physical checks while they talked about maternity leave and when it was best to give up work and how Nora could get a letter to say she needed to stop working at thirty-eight weeks. Ingrid addressed these questions, stopping to smile as she read the notes in Nora's pregnancy folder saying the baby weighed approximately 2.2kgs but still had plenty of time to grow, and they would get her off work when she wanted to stop. Ingrid wove everyday conversation about trying to get pregnant and the bureaucratic nuisances of organising maternity leave with a medical consultation. The consultation was half an hour long and they spent more time talking about issues outside of the medical check than about the examination itself. I frequently observed this. Here it is evident that comfort, sympathy and emotional responses were enfolded into a physical, biomedical check-up. More than just asking how Nora was, Ingrid relayed accounts that offered her client glimpses into her life outside of the midwifery practice. 'Familiarity' was being made as Ingrid spoke to Nora about particular 'banal' aspects of life alongside doing the familiar, comforting antenatal check-up. Therefore, the grounded persona of the midwife, talking in calm, everyday ways and showing an interest in her client's life, outside the pregnancy (a version of attention), produced a sense of 'familiarity'. Familiarity as a method used by midwives offers further insight into their work of normalising pregnancy and birth.

The midwives made a point of making women as comfortable as possible with small gestures, such as when, in the middle of winter, Beth warmed the gel used for the Doppler. The other midwives would put a towel on the heater so that women who had to remove their trousers, were able to stay warm, when the towel was put on them. Women who were feeling particularly tired or uncomfortable often lay on the exam table throughout the consultation, so they were able to be off their feet, and midwives would lean against the table, sympathising with their ailments. The midwives produced a relaxed rhythm for consultations.

Like Alex and Ingrid, Bridget had methods for making consultations relaxed, 'personal' and informal. Tim and Kirsten were expecting their first baby and were excited at the prospect of having a home birth. Bridget playfully scolded Tim that it was his job to organise the food, drinks and pool for Kirsten's birth. Kirsten was officially at 'term' (thirty-seven weeks onwards) and so while it could still be a while before labour began, Bridget instructed them on when to call if labour started and when not to, saying 'if its 3am and very mild, you should go back to sleep, that's best for everyone!' But if it was urgent or they were concerned, they should call rather than send a message as Bridget might not wake up to the soft sound of a message alert on her phone. Bridget sat in a relaxed manner, her one leg under the other, sipping water as Kirsten described people's negative or incredulous reactions to her having a home birth.

Indeed, Kirsten's decision to birth at home is considered an inappropriate stance and is evidence of the extent to which pregnancy and birth have been medicalised in South Africa. It is also illustrative of the ways in which pregnancy is indeed medicalised and understood as an event requiring hospitalisation.

Bridget offset this, working directly from her model of birth, that birth is overly medicalised. She said it was better not to tell people if possible: Kirsten had made an informed choice and Bridget felt she should trust that, not worrying what others thought. Like Marie, Kirsten knew her midwife's stance on safety and how she fronted safety and she was offered support to birth in a way regarded as 'irresponsible' by the medicalised fraternity. Bridget's support offset ideas of danger and irresponsibility by affirming the work of making an 'informed choice' as well as Bridget's constant assurances of safety.

Bridget's body language and way of sitting offered a 'relaxed', comfortable bodily comportment. Being available to Kirsten and relaying the 'ordinary' details of sleeping through phone messages worked to produce familiarity. Bridget's spoken and bodily responses offered the 'familiarity' and normality that Kirsten needed in light of her unusual birth choice. Her midwife was appropriately familiar (they knew each other) for an experience that was considered a 'normal' event. Thus, 'familiarity' was constructed by spending time talking (highlighting the importance of the thirty-minute and one-hour consultations which frequently went overtime) and talking about the everyday, in a particular tone of 'groundedness'.

'Familiarity' and 'groundedness' as relations of responsiveness speak to a desire for connection, availability and accompaniment.

Indeed, Alfonso Lingis (2003: 38) reflects in his meditation on trust that trust is presocial and pre-contractual, it is something that is within, that exists. It is beyond words and thinking; we do trust. Tim Ingold's (2000: 70) phenomenological account of trust in the context of environments illustrates trust as an embodied experience, as a relation of sharing. These notions of trust offer an insight into the work of familiarity and groundedness as accompanying work and practice based relations. The work of weaving conversations, comfort and empathy into a medical consultation are relationally orientated practices which highlight the embodied, practice orientated aspects of emotional work: care work is about responding to another (Lingis 2003).

Trust: Constructing Trust as a Relation of Care

The work of creating trust is embedded in how midwives create a sense of 'groundedness' and 'familiarity'. Trust is part of the emotional work women anticipated as they planned their pregnancy and care; here I describe the relation of trust as a mode of attentiveness and responsiveness and a skill-based practice co-created by those in my study. In doing this, I am able to engage in a discussion on the relations between attentiveness and responsiveness in the ethics of care. Below, I describe an interaction that demonstrates and reiterates the makings of trust.

Rachel, the patient safety officer whom we met in the introduction, drew from her professional experience and described how obstetric-led births rely on hospital midwives in the early labour stages. She felt that they were not well equipped; because they were managing more than one person, they could miss important findings in their checks. She said:

> Before I got to know Bridget, and built a trust relationship with her, I knew I needed the best midwife, who could pick up complications cos I was focussed all on the complications, she needed to be extremely well trained, knowledgeable, pick up the complications because that's what I'm exposed to all the time.
>
> It was me fighting for what I wanted versus, what I, who I am and the rational side of me. [I see] every single case of cerebral hypoxia where a mom has been hurt, baby has been hurt; these cross my desk on a daily basis. So every time a bladder is nicked in a C-section or a women dies from post-partum haemorrhage, you get a pulmonary

> embolism from a deep vein thrombosis, that's my everyday reality, and I thought, that by choosing the best midwife, who knows her stuff the best, I would get the best birthing experience, the safest birthing experience.

Rachel connects 'the best' birthing experience with safety. Even though she appears to emphasise safety above other concerns, her need for a particular attention was revealed in her later criticism of the practice of in-house (hospital-provided) midwives having to manage more than one woman in labour. Rachel, like Marie, wanted safety but she framed all the attention she desired in terms of safety rather than 'personality' and 'knowing' Bridget. Trust was constituted as a combination of being offered support, companionship and 'knowing' the midwife in conjunction with safety and knowing the limits (see Chapter 3). Marie, Gill and Jeanne's accounts affirm this. There were a series of relations at work in the consultations. Familiarity was constructed in the language of the everyday, sympathy and groundedness. Safety and support were interwoven to produce trust. Familiarity and trust, in combination, constituted intimacy in care work.

Navigating Birthing Relations: Intimacy

The crafting of intimacy in care work took time. The foundations for intimacy were built on the relations of trust, familiarity and groundedness. The attentions and experiences women in my study hoped for were provided in intimacy. Women felt they 'knew' their midwives in several important ways. They knew them as carers offering safety and support. They also knew them as 'friends' – people who spoke about the everyday, who took an interest in their lives, revealed parts of their personality (or so it appeared) and offered sympathy and accompaniment. Indeed, Lynne described her midwives as 'expert-aunts': women she could trust with her safety and whom she was able to sit down and 'have a cup of tea with'. The midwife as an 'intimate' carer is critical to their work.

In opening a conversation on intimacy, I look to Brigitte Jordan's (1978: 10) account of birth. She suggests that birth is difficult to study because it consists to a large degree of non-public intimacy involving bodily functions and displays. The same can be said of the antenatal consultation in which bodily functions such as urine and blood pressure are checked and bodies are exposed.

While birth may be described as 'an intimate event', that does not necessarily mean there is intimacy present. The women in my study insisted on intimacy as a relation, being present in consultations. Elizabeth Grosz (2003:125) writes: 'it is in intimate and/or nurturing relations that we are encouraged not just to look but also to show, not just to look, but also to induce a touching. Nakedness is a lure to intimacy and proximity because it invites the other's care and solicitude'.

Grosz highlights the deeply relational, co-produced elements of intimacy. The attentions women desired in light of Grosz' reflections can perhaps be understood as 'invitations' to respond in intimate ways: constructing trust and familiarity were therefore the responses the midwives offered in this thoroughly social relation. Yet it is important not to romanticise an intimacy that was, after all, professional. Cheryl Hunter (2012) describes doula care in the US as providing what she calls one-sided intimacy. By this she means that clients may feel a connection with their carer but the carer does not need to feel that connection too. This is true of the midwives in my study: they offered a service, not friendship. Yet intimacy was constituted in relations. It may have been felt only by clients, but it was relationally produced. This presents a paradox: how can a relation be built purposefully between two people but only experienced in a particular way by one of them?

This paradox offers, if you will, an ethics of self-care. In order to elaborate on this point, a discussion on the ethics of care and the virtues of attentiveness and responsiveness, as described by Tronto (1993), is necessary. Care receivers, in the model of responsiveness, are imbued with agency. It is the responsibility of a care receiver to respond to what is being offered as care, assessing the forms care takes (Tronto 1993: 107, 108). Relationship is key here, and ideally care giver and receiver are both respected so that care becomes a negotiation. Yet responsiveness is, for Tronto (1993: 107), the final phase of caring. Indeed, care moves through stages of caring about, taking care of, care giving and finally, care receiving.

My findings suggest that care was anticipated in particular ways at the very beginning of the midwife-client relationship. More than this, as clients, women expected a version of care which they relayed to me as 'why they chose a midwife' – the midwife represented both a version of birth and a particular kind of care. Responses (how midwives would respond and provide care) were therefore known before care was complete and this finding offers an account of the relationality and interwoven quality of the phases of care. It also affirms Clara Han's (2012: 24) point that care can be defined as 'a problem rather than a given' requiring everyday attentions and responsiveness to others. As Livingston (2012) writes, care is deeply social, and those in care relationships can be called partners in care. Therefore the relational qualities of building intimacy and responsiveness suggest that because women desired responsiveness from the beginnings of care, they directed birthing relations as practices of self-care. Thus intimacy could be one-sided but relational as a mode of self-care instantiated by women's care wishes.

An Ethics of Self-Care in Birthing Relations

Here, I open the discussion on the relationality of care phases and care of the self. First, it is necessary to define how I use this phrase. Foucault, who noted that modern medicine is a technology of power, objectifying the body in order to control it, writes:

> Medicine was not conceived simply as a technique of intervention, relying, in cases of illness, on remedies and operations. It was also supposed to define, in the form of a corpus of knowledge and rules, a way of living, a reflective mode of relation to oneself, to one's body, to one's food, to wakefulness and sleep, to the various activities, and to the environment. Medicine was expected to propose, in the form of regimen, a voluntary and rational structure of conduct'. (Foucault 1986: 99–100)

The individual, assumed to be an autonomous subject in the cultivation of the self, engages techniques and practices of self-care. As Han (2012: 5) writes, however, '"self-care" and "self-responsibility" assume a self that is sovereign, morally autonomous and transposed'. As I have noted in Chapter 1, however, the people in my study were those for whom liberal democracy works. Indeed, they engaged care, 'choice' and 'responsibility' as liberal subjects and enjoyed the benefits of privilege. Thus, a 'responsibilisation' of care was assumed by those in my study and I suggest that birthing relations operate as modes for self-care (Zigon 2008).

If you will, the 'failure' that comes with 'poor' planning and decision making in a privileged setting of choice (Shaw 2002) was offset by choosing a carer and care that offered a scenario in which, irrelevant of how the birth unfolded, it would still be experienced as 'positive'. The work of planning and having a particular version of birth led to the makings of the self, women and mothers. Women in my study took this a step further: they anticipated and determined the care they would receive. That care, upholding a cultural model of birth deemed natural, defined them as 'good mothers' and 'women good at being mothers' (Zigon 2008). Care as practised by others towards women, also therefore constructed self-care as women protected themselves from 'poor' planning and feeling 'uninvolved' in their pregnancies. Doing work that made the 'good mother' necessitated care and intimacy and as a mode of responsiveness, carefully co-constructed, it emerged between women and their midwives.

As we have seen, my informants elaborated their wishes and imaginings of care, formalising them in their broader planning approach to pregnancy and concretising them in birth plans. Women fashioned the self in the pain stories they told. Here, in the construction of birthing relations, these approaches to pregnancy and the self came to constitute an ethics of self-care.

Intimacy and Birthing: Midwives at Work

I have shown how intimacy is made over the course of pregnancy. As trust and familiarity were built during consultations, these relations would be experienced as important elements when it came to labour and birth. Below, I describe Lucy's birth, the first I witnessed.

It was already a hot Sunday in March when I received a message that morning from Lucy saying she was in early labour so I should keep my day 'open'. She had impatiently awaited labour and her husband, James, appeared to be showing some strain when they came into their last consultation, rolling his eyes at me and Bridget when Lucy went to the bathroom to give a urine sample.

I was therefore happy for her that she had gone into labour shortly after reaching forty weeks gestation. Later on Sunday afternoon I received messages from Lucy and Bridget saying I should come over to Lucy's house, and that Bridget would shortly be there. When I got there, James was rushing, filling the birth pool, sweating as he carried buckets of water into the bedroom, as the day had steadily become hotter. Lucy's labour was speeding up, and filling the pool from the hosepipe was not filling the pool quickly enough. Bridget told me to go and say hello to Lucy who was leaning against the bed, her head pressed between her arms. The room was dark and warm, with all the curtains drawn. We said hello and Bridget joined us, kneeling next to Lucy, holding her hand and stroking her back as she whispered in her ear that she was 'doing really well'. About ten minutes later Lucy hurriedly told us she needed to push so Bridget told her she could get in the pool. Quickly Lucy's composure changed. She suddenly seemed panicked, grunting suddenly, and told Bridget between contractions that she needed her to 'tell her when and how to push'. Bridget, sitting at the side of the pool, close to Lucy's head with a torch secured around her forehead, explained that as soon as she wanted to push, she should do so. Bridget placed her Doppler in the water and listened to the baby's heartbeat and soon Lucy indicated she was having a contraction and she began pushing. Bridget told her how to breathe short breaths, panting like a dog as the head began to emerge, but as she did so, there was meconium in the pool.[6] Bridget firmly but gently told Lucy to stand up quickly, to get her pelvis out of the water. James assisted her and held her up as she pushed again. The baby's head emerged. Bridget jumped into the pool to 'catch' the baby. Bridget asked her assistant to hand over the suction equipment so they could clear the baby's mouth. He soon breathed and Lucy was able to get back in the pool, her son resting against her chest.

Everyone breathed a sigh of relief; the birth had unfolded quickly – Bridget, her assistant and I had not been there more than twenty minutes – and it had felt rushed. Bridget checked the baby and smiled at Lucy telling her she had 'done great'. After that, James took his son and Lucy expelled the placenta. She soon got out of the bath and Bridget sat with her on the bed. Lucy kept saying 'thank you Bridget, I didn't know how to do it without you!' She said she had no idea how to push, despite having done it before, and she needed Bridget's guidance. As Bridget checked Lucy's perineum (the skin between the vagina and anus that can be torn in childbirth), Lucy held her baby and began feeding him. Once Lucy had rested for half an hour, and her midwife had checked the placenta, Bridget asked her if she could try and urinate (it is often hard to urinate after birth) and 'get cleaned up'. Lucy was so shaky, tired and sore that Bridget helped her to the bathroom, holding her up, and assisted her as she showered, bending down, drying her legs, as Lucy could not bend down herself. We all left soon after this, leaving Lucy and her baby settled in bed, happy and serene. When I got home, reflecting on all I had witnessed, I wrote the following:

> The work of a midwife is very humble, 'on the ground work'. I sat watching the midwife clean up after the birth, drying new mother's body, checking through the placenta for any missing bits (the placenta is beautiful – it looks just like a tree of life), stitching a woman's body and then sorting through needles and wires to discard as medical waste (the needles need to be separated from the waste so cleaners do not hurt themselves). There is nothing fancy or sophisticated or flashy about midwives' work: the room after birth smells strongly of blood, the floor is a mess, there is excrement, mucus, blood, placenta – the room is heavy with a rawness of life – and yet the woman with her new baby is glowing, beautiful.

Lucy's birth offers an insight into the embodied work of trust, familiarity and intimacy. As Bridget, her assistant and I sipped tea and water in Lucy's living room, while she rested in bed, there was an easy familiarity in place. Such work had been initiated months ago. Indeed, as MacDonald (2007: 152) notes, natural home births are actively produced. Dark lighting with candles, a warm space with soft music are stereotypes of home births for good reason: home birth looks like this. In fact, this was a common scene in the hospital births I witnessed too, except that fairy lights were used instead of candles. Intimacy was built in consultations but it was also enacted in specific renderings in space. Home, or a home-away-from-home in hospital, is therefore symbolic of intimacy and familiarity. The midwife, having constructed birthing relations, is able to step into such a space. Yet there were limits to care work.

Intimacies and Limits

Cheryl Hunter (2012) notes that intimacy shifts the way in which care is experienced. She suggests intimacy is a combination of familiarity, attending to small touches and taking on a role as a 'mother figure'. It is important and necessary to recognise that despite the attentions and experiences of connection and intimacy my informants envisaged, care work and the client-midwife relationship are limited in two ways: limited in the sharing of intimacy and limited in time. Below, Bridget describes the work that goes into assessing and working with her clients.

> So for me I'm trying to understand where she is at, where she's coming from, what are her unique drivers, fears, circumstances that can affect her birthing. What she needs from me: some people need very

> overt, very direct nurturing and bossing, others, you know, don't. Those are the ones that have very quick appointments. And they'll contact me if there is something and then there are my others, I call (laughs) 'frequent phoners'. Every now and then you get one that often emails and messages, more 'intensive'. In the end though, I want them to feel empowered, so that no matter the outcome, they feel it was a consultative process and they made decisions along the way, they didn't feel like they were pushed into things, cheated out of an experience. They're not looking back traumatised or unsure of interventions being necessary, rather enjoying the experience.

Bridget expressed a need to account for each of her client's 'drivers' and she recognises that the women in her care have care needs that they expect her to provide. Over and above her sometimes having to work with 'intensive' or 'high-maintenance' clients was a wish to empower her clients with a positive birth experience. Her account of care presents us with a view of the ways in which midwives worked. Marie and Gill understood themselves as knowing their midwife's personality and vice versa but Bridget's comment suggests that her work in 'getting to know' clients was about learning how to care for them and offer them what they needed in antenatal care and support. She did this by creating familiarity. She does not, however, speak about how her clients know her because despite Gill's reflection, clients do not know their midwives outside their professional role. While Bridget made it clear that her clients should communicate with her, she offers a glimpse into her perspective: women who called frequently were not 'good friends', they were 'high-maintenance clients'. The midwives worked through 'difficult' situations of 'over-phoning' by assisting women during pregnancy and labour but then making it clear care was finished with the six-week postnatal check being the last encounter. There are therefore limits to care work.

The limits of care ask what constitutes 'enough'. What is meant by 'enough' intimacy and 'enough' 'emotional care' is addressed in the ways in which 'personality' and 'knowing' the midwife are framed in terms of familiarity. Knowing the midwife 'a little' or 'just enough' or as Marie commented, wanting her carer to be 'strong enough', describe the parameters of care relations. As a concept, 'intimacy' operates as a marker of what is revealed in a care relationship and by whom, and 'enough' is a tool for thinking about and crafting the depths of familiarity, trust and intimacy and modulates the depth and breadth of care work and its associated relations.

Time and Its Limits in Midwifery Care

I have presented an account of how birthing relations are made and therefore an ethnographic account would not be complete without a description of the unmaking of relations. The end of care warrants attention. After birth, women were visited in their homes four days postnatally. After that they had one more consultation with their midwife in which stitches were checked and bellies felt, establishing that the uterus had shrunk back to its non-pregnant size. After this, midwives wished women well and gave them a hug. The relation was over. My informants expressed feeling sadness at this realisation, describing how their midwife had been present at the birth of their child but was suddenly absent. One woman in my study expressed sadness at the end of her time with the midwives, saying she felt her midwife was 'cheating' on her, in relation to the midwives helping other women after her.

Midwives sometimes felt the same way. Ingrid described how she enjoyed some women so much that it was 'a little sad' when the pregnancy was over, but continuing a relationship was impossible because midwives would become advisors to women indefinitely. Their services had been rendered and the work was over. Tanya told me that she used to have annual 'teas' for all their clients but it became a space where women asked her advice and sought care in a similar fashion to the antenatal consultations. Tanya and Ingrid recognised the need to end care well and definitely. The potential for slippages and blurring boundaries was too great. Each midwife was able to relay a story of a woman who took advantage of their care, calling too often post-birth and expecting more house calls. The use of intimacy in creating relations for birthing had a drawback: intimacy is built up. Starkly removing intimacy is difficult.

Han's account of care as a problem perhaps best illustrates the end of care. Taking care as a problem seriously, it is possible to recognise the ways in which care happens. In her account of informal care, people fail one another, care does not always work and people do not always respond to care (2012: 29). In my study, care was bought and that in some ways made care more straightforward; it was a service purchased for a designated time. Having said that, I have shown how birthing relations were far more complex than a service definition of care suggests. Indeed, care was co-constructed. Care as a problem in this context offers an insight into how emotional work and relations can be constructed as a service with an inevitable end. The inevitable end of intimacy in birthing relations is perhaps a failure of this care model, even if it is a necessary failure. The inherently social, relational aspects of care present the end of care with unsatisfactory finality. That is indeed the limit of the care midwives offered. Their work relied on intimacy but intimacy was finite.

Conclusion

Following Patti Henderson (2012) who writes how touch is a way that intimate, social worlds are shared and materialise, I proposed that the midwives could not care without intimacy enfolding their work: their hands felt wellness, provided support and caught babies, their clients demanded it and this produced challenges at the end of care. Lauren Berlant (1998) articulates the ways in which intimate events are predicated on institutions of intimacy. Intimacy, she writes, builds worlds. By destabilising intimacy and its spaces, Berlant (1998: 283) insists that the conflation of intimacy and 'having a life' instantiates a fantasy that private life is real in relation to collective life. In social worlds of flux and disorder, the project of intimacy seeks to stabilise a small pocket of life: the sanctuary of home, love and family. Modernist imperatives that establish binaries of work and personal life stabilise the personal, making collective life tolerable.

Berlant's account compels us to recognise the social, collective quality of intimacy. The articulation of a need for intimacy in midwives' care giving offers ways of thinking through care. Care demonstrates how intimacy and collective life are deeply entangled. To follow Henderson (2012: 102), women and midwives were engaged in repertoires of relatedness beyond typical family and kin definitions. The embodied work of care by midwives and the private rhythms of pregnant women that were shared with midwives as social rhythms came to bear on a fleshy, familial, bodily version of care. Yet in my study, intimacy in antenatal care needed to be purchased and was therefore available to very few. Self-care as a practice enacted in birthing relations needed to be bought. This fact offers a reflection on liberal subjectivity and modern reproductive lives. The critiques of the notion of the autonomous subject, etched into the precarity of being 'poor', are perhaps also relevant to those for whom liberal democratic life works. Indeed, the individual subject, in attempts to offset isolation and alienation, must insist on relational, intimate care work with capital.

The latter point draws attention to how birth and parenting are understood as activities to be undertaken by individuals or in a dyad, rather than in an extended network. Women sought out and purchased relations in the form of midwife care. Particular bodies were produced within this model, reproduced in the version of care available to an elite few. This draws us back to the anticipation of attention, foregrounded earlier in the chapter. It reveals how modern middle-class South African women, wanting an experience and attention that necessitated emotional responses and intimacy, were indeed asking to be seen and responded to in 'emotional work' and obtaining that entailed a consumer-driven approach to intimacy. This supports Tronto's (1993) point that boundaries between political and moral worlds, the public and private spaces of care exist, problematically so. Sevenhuijsen (1998) calls for care practices to be integrated into concepts of citizenship. My study has shown the privilege of access to care, but also how the need for relations of intimacy, accompaniment, attentiveness and responsiveness have been constructed and reproduced by (largely white) economically elite citizens, as a formalised service that offers collective, intimate materialisations of birthing relations, where these relations are not a given.

Notes

1. During fieldwork the practice had some changes made: the walls were painted light grey, pictures were mounted of women in labour and their newly born babies, and the waiting room had pictures of each midwife placed near the fireplace with a caption about her, her children and her qualifications.
2. I return to the idea of 'an experience' in more detail later on in the chapter.
3. It is understood in emerging research on vaginal birth that vaginally born babies initiate breastfeeding quicker than C-section delivered babies and that breastfeeding complications are more likely with the latter.
4. Indeed, kinship definitions have been stretched as donors, surrogates and IVF become pathways to parenthood. Babies have come to be known as semi-individuated beings known in ways made available via technologies such as the Doppler, ultrasound and amniocentesis.
5. It is interesting that Young's work, written over thirty years ago, still applies to expectant parents' experiences. This speaks, perhaps, to the medicalisation of birth in South Africa at present.

6. A dark green substance that is the baby's first stool in utero. Meconium is normally stored in the infant's intestines until after birth, but sometimes (often in response to foetal distress and hypoxia) it is expelled into the amniotic fluid prior to birth, or during labour. If the baby then inhales the contaminated fluid, respiratory problems may occur. If a baby is in distress, it is more inclined to take a first breath in water, making a water birth unsafe.

Conclusion

Care as a Problem, Care's Limits

Ingrid spoke to me one morning in between consultations about the conversations that were happening between the midwives about the length of time of consultations. Some of the midwives felt the half-hour long follow-up appointments were not long enough for their clients as they frequently ran 'over-time'. I knew this was true, regularly observing two of the midwives run ten to twenty minutes late. Ingrid, having trained in the United Kingdom, felt the increased consultation time was unnecessary, commenting that 'this really is the Rolls-Royce of care'. Her comment and the discussion it referred to typifies the sets of expectations, versions of attention and accompaniment that shaped the care independent midwives provided as they offered women time. They gave women their time as they listened to them and spent hours supporting them in labour and caring for them in the weeks post-birth.

Such aspirations made me wonder if the care I was observing was a practise to be emulated in wider South African health care or if it was simply another kind of entitlement available only to the rich (and white). Later that day, Ingrid comforted Molly, who was worrying about giving birth, about how she would manage with a new baby and about post-partum depression. A gentle hand on a shoulder, the reassuring check of her baby's wellbeing and a conversation about support in labour allowed Molly to leave the consultation with a lighter heart and mind. The interaction presents the difficulty of care that is 'good', 'well-intended' and genuine but deeply privileged. It continues to sit uncomfortably.

Clara Han (2012), in her exploration of care as a problem, asks how anthropology can attend to the ways in which people can simultaneously be present to and fail one another. Han (2012) describes the interwoven qualities and the different registers of debt that mark life for the Chilean poor. She reminds us of the connections between broader moral and social debts to those who suffered under the Pinochet dictatorship and the debts of those in close quarters: family, neighbours and friends. Amid day-to-day struggles, the people in her study find ways to care for one another, sensitively and discreetly offering care and support in ways that attempt to offset the humiliating provision of state services. She asks us to be open to possibility and contingency, and argues that in paying attention to specific lives, the traces and reworkings of conventions and norms are made visible. Such a method enables Han to see care that might otherwise go unnoticed. Care in this context might in fact not be recognised as care at all, as it is enmeshed in the daily struggles of shame, stigma and precarity. Care is rightly presented as a problem in Han's account.

While not the same as Chile, the South African context bears striking resemblances to it. A history of enormous injustice and human rights abuses alongside a capitalist economy continues to make life 'raw' (Ross 2010). The question of being present to and concurrently failing one another can be engaged on a small scale, for the group of women in my study. Midwives presented intimate versions of care, but also presented limits, and final ends to their care work that were abrupt, stark and left women feeling 'cheated on' by their midwife as time worked to end relations and bring new babies into the world.

Han's enquiry can also be brought to bear more broadly on South African social life and its inequalities, where the work of the midwives presents care as a different kind of problem. A model of care that emulates and instantiates reassurance, trust, intimacy and connection also perpetuates ideas and options of choice and entitlement for the rich. South Africa's care worlds are deeply stratified; for liberal subjects, for whom resources, and economic and social structures are available, these structures have allowed for choice and 'best birthing' practices. For others, who lack those resources and who 'failed' in South Africa's democracy to reach the potential of a self-made person, pregnancy and birth are still centred on life, death and survival, not choice (Povinelli 2002).

For women in my study, choice was the axis upon which birthing was approached and choice was understood as inevitable and as a 'right'. Privilege, for Povinelli (2007: 80), is a form of amnesia 'that many people consider life as something that can be counted on, at least for a certain length of time, for long enough to be able to forget about its limited nature'. Women in my study and their midwives were able to take life for granted – a life of resources and medical insurance – and that their babies would be born safe, well and alive.

South Africa's model of capitalism, initially enacted in racial form, now practised in the form of a neo-liberal economy, continues to make certain kinds of life possible for some and not others (Ross 2010). The possibilities presented to middle-class white women as they navigated birthing choices and 'best birth practices' enabled particular experiences, births and futures. At stake in the work of the midwives was the reproduction of privilege.

Glenn (1994), in her paper on reproductive labour and its relationship to race, draws attention to the connection between reproductive labour and privilege. She shows how historically speaking, women have tended to take on the majority of the maintenance of family and household – preparing food, caring for children and maintaining social and family ties – an invisible form of labour that allows, typically, for men to benefit directly and indirectly from it. Direct benefits include having to contribute less to households and their maintenance. Indirectly, and significantly, people not doing reproductive labour are able to focus attention on paid employment. A gender-based division in reproductive labour establishes gendered divisions in the work place. Such an arrangement draws attention to the relationship between production and reproduction, and gendered privileges in both realms (Glenn 1992). There is a relationship between reproductive work and privilege, an association that feminists have highlighted. Glenn goes further to demonstrate the ways in which race has impacted availabilities to work but has largely been ignored in the realm of reproductive labour. This point, alongside Fraser's (1997) argument that material inequalities and misrecognition need to be differentiated, demonstrates that there are connections between race, reproductive labour and privilege. Critically, for the women in my study, reproduction was also connected to desires for recognition.

Feminist discourse has described the connections between reproductive labour and gendered forms of privilege. The racial divisions of such forms of labour and privilege have also been described (Xaba 2017). Privilege takes form in different ways to the usual gendered instantiations in this study. Privilege was about having access to care that needed to be paid for rather than provided by the state. For women who were able to plan and make 'choices' about their care and births, privilege made this choice appear possible and choices needed meanings that women expressed in modes of planning and orientations to pain. The recognition that women sought, as they attempted to make meaning from birthing a specific way – naturally – produced specific attentions, availabilities and kinds of care. Births occurred and were experienced in ways that only an elite few could access and experience. The connections between privilege and reproductive work were directly linked to race and the recognition women sought. The fact of being able to make a choice, and the choices women made, produced a series of affects available as an elite resource.

This study has focused attention on a group of women who understand their care as inevitable, and who draw on certain feminist discourses, as a 'right'. They purchased their own private birthing experience in a deliberate and planned act of 'resistance', defying expectations and norms of giving birth in a controlled and alienating private health care environment. Their privilege was many things, including ignorance. The fact of being able to access private care, and find it lacking, reflects a privilege and access to care that is extraordinary in South Africa.

Where, with whom and how one birthed were all shaped by the amount of capital a family was able to access and, largely, how they were categorised during Apartheid. Not only did this offer the women in my study 'choice', it also gave them 'purchasing power' – if they did not like a service, they could take their money elsewhere. Care was modulated in accordance with these sets of expectations and intimate, familial care was purchased by an elite group of South African citizens. In South Africa, as I have shown, inequality in care and available resources is instantiated and reproduced via class, race and privilege. Because privilege is largely still racially defined and enacted, the reproduction of privilege is the reproduction of race in South Africa.

For economically elite citizens, the political economy of the distribution of services ensured they were able to access the care and births of their choice. They were also, by demanding familial intimacy in care work as a service, able to insist on a particular kind of affect. Therefore, the political economy of the distribution of resources was not just about white families being able to access certain health care services, it was also about the political economy of the distribution of affect.

The connections between privilege, race and reproduction are rendered easily visible at each birth witnessed and discussed in this study. Care continues to work both as an imperative and as a problem. In the lives of each woman using a midwife, care was about being recognised, seen and heard. Care was about instantiating a series of affects that are found lacking in a liberal economy in which broader social networks of care and support are absent. Care is also about reproducing race in a context where privilege is aligned with the colour of one's skin and the potential afforded to some and not others. Care is asked to do a great deal. As midwives were present for their clients and women experienced 'positive' births, other South African women did not. The care worlds of South Africans are disparate in many ways but those worlds are also connected. The forms of care I witnessed were gentle and intimate; they also formed part of a broader set of structures that alienate, exclude and reproduce racial inequalities. The fragility of humanness seen in delicate care work is founded on and replicates a model of exclusion. The trouble with care is that we cannot do without it; but for some, the care they call for means that others must continue to do without: care in this context has limits but it also limits others.

Appendix

Hypnobirthing Terms – from *HypnoBirthing: The Mongan Method*

Medicalised language	**Hypnobirthing language**
Birth canal	Birth path
Bloody show	Birth show
Catch the baby	Receive the baby
Coach	Birth companion
Complications	Special circumstances
Contraction	Uterine surge or wave
Deliver/delivery	Birth/birthing
Due date	Birthing time/month
Effacing/dilating	Thinning/opening
Foetus	Pre-born/unborn baby
Mucous plug	Uterine seal
Pain or contractions	Pressure/sensation/tightening
Primip/Multip	First-/second-time mom
Pushing	Birth breathing
Transition	Near completion/near complete
Water breaking/rupturing	Membranes releasing

Glossary

Amniotic fluid – fluid that surrounds the baby in utero.

Birthing pool – inflatable pool used by labouring women as a pain relief method. The pool is filled with 37°C water (anything hotter than body temperature can cause foetal distress), submerging the labouring women's body.

Birthing stool – a stool with a semi-circular opening in the centre used in labour to help facilitate upright birthing positions. The stool enables a supported squatting position.

Booking consultation – the first consultation with a midwife in which medical history taking is done along with blood work. Approximately one hour long.

Breech presentation – the position of a baby in which the feet or buttocks appear first during birth.

Caesarean section (C-section) – a surgical operation for delivering a baby by cutting through the wall of the mother's abdomen.

Cardiotocography (CTG) – measures the baby's heart rate. At the same time it also monitors the contractions in the uterus. CTG is used both before birth (antenatally) and during labour, to monitor the baby for any signs of distress.

Cephalic presentation – the position of a baby in which the head appears first during birth.

Cervix – the opening of the uterus.

Chat visit – a first meeting and information session in which women have not booked with the midwife yet but are able to find out about midwife-led care and the midwife.

Cephalopelvic Disproportion (CPD) – when the baby's head does not fit through the pelvis.

Delayed cord clamping –a birth practice where the umbilical cord is not clamped or cut until after pulsations have ceased, or until after the placenta is delivered.

Dilation – the opening of the cervix (measured in centimetres – 10cm being fully dilated), and effacement, the thinning of the cervix (measured in percentage) during labour. This is considered the first stage of labour and in primigravida women can take several hours.

Doppler – a hand held device used to listen to a baby's heartbeat and hence, assess wellness.

Engaged – in the last weeks, sometime before birth, the baby's head can move down into the pelvis. When this happens, the baby is said to be 'engaged'.

Epidural – epidural anaesthesia is a regional anaesthesia that blocks pain in a particular region of the body. The goal of an epidural is to provide analgesia, or pain relief, rather than anaesthesia, which leads to total lack of feeling. Epidurals block the nerve impulses from the lower spinal segments.

Episiotomy – a surgical cut in the muscular area between the vagina and the anus (the area called the perineum) made just before delivery to enlarge the vaginal opening.

Estimated Due Date (EDD) – the date a baby is estimated to arrive on the basis of the last period date and early scans.

External Cephalic Version (ECV) – a procedure used to turn a baby from a breech position or side-lying (transverse) position into a head-down (vertex) position before labour begins.

Footling breech – a footling breech is when one or both of the baby's feet are born first instead of the bottom.

Forceps – a health care provider applies forceps, an instrument shaped like a pair of large spoons or salad tongs, to the baby's head to help assist delivery.

Home Birth after Caesarean Section (HBAC) – attempting to have a vaginal birth at home after one or more C-sections.

Induction – contractions can be started by inserting a pessary or gel into the vagina, and sometimes both are used. Induction of labour may take a while, particularly if the cervix (the neck of the uterus) needs to be softened with pessaries or gels. Sometimes a hormone drip (Syntocinon/Pitocin) is needed to speed up the labour.

Infant Mortality Rate (IMR) – the number of deaths of infants under one year old per 1,000 live births. This rate is often used as an indicator of the level of health in a country. South Africa's is 29 per 1000 and WHO regards 18 per 1000 as acceptable (World Bank 2015).

Intrauterine Insemination (IUI) – artificial form of insemination where a syringe or catheter is used to insert sperm into the uterus.

Intervention free – a birth that has no surgical or medical intervention in the form of analgesia, induction, episiotomy, forceps or ventouse delivery, and C-section.

Kangaroo Mother Care (KMC) – immediate skin-to-skin contact at birth, with exclusive breastfeeding and supporting the mother-child dyad. Particularly beneficial to premature babies.

Labour – Active – the stage of labour in which the cervix is dilated to 5cm+ and contractions are approximately one minute long with three in ten minutes.

Maternal Mortality Rate (MMR) – the annual number of female deaths per 100,000 live births from any cause related to or aggravated by pregnancy or its management (excluding accidental or incidental causes). South Africa's current MMR is 138 per 100,000 births (WHO 2017).

Meconium – a dark green substance that is the baby's first stool in utero. Meconium is normally stored in the infant's intestines until after birth, but sometimes (often in response to foetal distress and hypoxia) it is expelled into the amniotic fluid prior to birth, or during labour.

Obstetric Cholestasis – a liver disorder that occurs where the normal flow of bile out of the liver is reduced. Labour generally needs to be induced so that the baby is born prior to the condition becoming dangerous to baby and woman.

Oxytocin – a hormone responsible for initiating labour and contractions.

Positions – Left Occipital Anterior – where the baby's head is down, with its back on the left side of the woman and its spine facing away from the woman's spine. The ideal birth position.

Positions – Left Occipital Posterior – where the baby's head is down, with its back on the left side of the woman and its spine against the woman's spine.

Positions – Right Occipital Anterior – where the baby's head is down, with its back on the right side of the woman and its spine facing away from the woman's spine.

Positions – Right Occipital Posterior – where the baby's head is down, with its back on the right side of the women and its spine against the woman's spine.

Primigravida – a woman who is pregnant for the first time.

Ruptured membranes – (ROM) or amniorrhexis is a term used during pregnancy to describe a rupture of the amniotic sac. Normally, it occurs spontaneously at full term either during or at the beginning of labour. Rupture of the membranes is known colloquially as 'breaking the water' or as one's 'water breaking.'

Stretch and Sweep – a stretch and sweep or membrane sweep is a relatively gentle way of trying to start labour. It sometimes initiates labour, reducing the risk of babies being born over the due date (forty-two weeks of pregnancy). The midwife puts a couple of lubricated, gloved fingers into the vagina and inserts their index finger into the opening of the cervix or neck of the uterus. They then use a circular movement to try to separate the membranes of the amniotic sac, containing the baby, from the cervix. This action releases hormones, called 'prostaglandins', which prepare the cervix for birth and initiates labour.

Syntocinon/Pitocin – a synthetic version of oxytocin, used to initiate labour.

Term/full term – the word used to describe a baby that has reached full growth, considered ready to be born. Term is from thirty-seven weeks gestation onwards.

Tracing – recording of the baby's heart rate for approximately thirty minutes in early labour or arrival at hospital to get a sense of the baby's wellbeing.

Transition – the cervix is dilated to 8cm+ and labour becomes intense with contractions coming very close together.

Transverse presentation – a baby lying sideways across the uterus and pelvic inlet.

Umbilical cord – a flexible cordlike structure containing blood vessels and attaching a baby to the placenta during gestation.

Urine Sample – used to assess bladder or kidney infections, diabetes, dehydration and preeclampsia by screening for high levels of sugars, proteins, ketones and bacteria. High levels of sugars may suggest gestational diabetes, which may develop around the twentieth week of pregnancy.

Vaginal Birth after Caesarean Section (VBAC) – attempting a vaginal birth after one or more C-sections.

Ventouse – also known as vacuum-assisted vaginal delivery or vacuum extraction (VE), a method to assist the delivery of a baby using a vacuum device. It is used in the second stage of labour if it has not progressed adequately. It may be an alternative to a forceps delivery and C-section.

References

Abrahams, N., R. Jewkes and Z. Mvo. 2001. 'Health Care-seeking Practices of Pregnant Women and the Role of Midwives in Cape Town, South Africa', *Journal of Midwifery and Women's Health* 46(4): 240–47.

Allen, Denise Roth. 2004. *Managing Motherhood Managing Risk: Fertility and Danger in West Central Tanzania.* Ann Arbor, MI: University of Michigan Press.

Asad, T. 2003. *Formations of the Secular: Christianity, Islam, Modernity.* Palo Alto, CA: Stanford University Press.

Avishai, O. 2007. 'Managing the Lactating Body: The Breastfeeding Project and Privileged Motherhood', *Qualia Sociologica* 30: 135–52.

Ayo, N. 2012. 'Understanding Health Promotion in a Neoliberal Climate and the Making of Health Conscious Citizens', *Critical Public Health* 22(1): 99–105.

Baier, A. 1981. 'Frankena and Hume on Points of View', *Monist: An International Quarterly Journal of a General Philosophical Inquiry* 64: 342–58.

Barthes, R. 1957 (1972). *Mythologies.* London: Paladin.

Bartky, S. 1982. 'Narcissism, Femininity and Alienation', *Social Theory and Practice* 8: 127–43.

Bastien, J. 1978. *Mountain of the Condor: Metaphor and Ritual in an Andean Ayllu.* St. Paul: West.

_____. 1985. 'Qollahuaya-Andean Body Concepts: A Topographical-Hydraulic Model of Physiology', *American Anthropology* 87: 595–611.

Becker, G. 2000. *The Elusive Embryo: How Women and Men Approach New Reproductive Technologies.* Berkeley: University of California Press.

Beck-Gernsheim, E. 1996. 'Risk and Self: Encounters and Responses'. In S. Lash and B. Szerszynski (eds), *Risk, Environment and Modernity: Towards a New Ecology*. London: Sage.

Berlant, L. 1998. 'Special Issue: Intimacy', *Critical Inquiry* 24(2): 281–88.

Berman, R. and D. Slobin. 1995. *Relating Events in Narrative: A Crosslinguistic Development Study.* Hillsdale, NJ: Erlbaum.

Berry, L., L. Biersteker, A. Dawes, L. Lake and C. Smith. 2013. *South African Child Gauge Report 2013*. Cape Town: University of Cape Town, Children's Institute.

Bertaux, D. and M. Kohli. 1984. 'The Life Story Approach: A Continental View', *Annual Review of Sociology* 10: 215–37.

Bessell, T., S. McDonald, C. Silagy, J. Anderson, J. Hiller and L. Sansom. 2002. 'Do Internet Interventions for Consumers Cause More Harm Than Good? A Systematic Review', *Health Expect* 5: 28–37.

Blum, L. 1999. *At the Breast: Ideologies of Breastfeeding and Motherhood in the Contemporary United States*. Boston, MA: Beacon Press.

Blustein, J. 1991. *Care and Commitment: Taking the Personal Point of View*. Oxford: Oxford University Press.

Boddy, J. 1988. 'Womb as Oasis: The Symbolic Context of Pharaonic Circumcision in Northern Sudan', *American Ethnologist* 9: 682–98.

Bosomworth, A. and J. Bettany-Saltikov. 2006. 'Just Take a Deep Breath: A Review to Compare the Effects of Spontaneous versus Directed Valsalva Pushing in the Second Stage of Labour on Maternal and Foetal Wellbeing'. *Midwifery Digest* 16(2): 157–166.

Bourdieu, P. 1977. *Outline of a Theory of Practice*. Cambridge: Cambridge University Press.

Bradshaw, D. and R. Dorrington.2012. 'Maternal Mortality Ratio – Trends in the Vital Registration Data', *South African Journalof Obstetrics and Gynaecology* 18: 38–42.

Brownridge, P. 1995. 'The Nature and Consequences of Childbirth Pain', *European Journal of Obstetrics and Gynaecology and Reproductive Biology* 59: 9–15.

Bryant, J., M. Porter, S. Tracy and E. Sullivan. 2007. 'Caesarean Birth: Consumption, Safety, Order, and Good Mothering', *Social Science and Medicine* 65(6): 1192–1201.

Burman, S. and P. Reynolds (eds). 1986. *Growing Up in a Divided Society*. Cape Town: David Philip.

Burtch, B. 1988. 'Midwifery and the State: The New Midwifery in Canada', in A. McLaren (ed.), *Gender and Society: Creating a Canadian Women's Sociology*. Toronto: Pitman.

Cavell, S. 1979. *The Claim of Reason: Wittgenstein, Skepticism, Morality, and Tragedy*. New York: Oxford University Press.

Chadwick, R. 2007. *Paradoxical Subjects: Women Telling Birth Stories*. Unpublished PhD dissertation, University of Cape Town.

_____. 2018. *Bodies that Birth: Revitalising Birth Politics*. London: Routledge.

Chadwick, R., D. Cooper and J. Harries. 2014. 'Narratives of Distress about Birth in South African Public Maternity Settings: A Qualitative Study', *Midwifery* 30: 862–68.

Chadwick, R. and D. Foster. 2013. 'Negotiating Risky Bodies: Childbirth and Constructions of Risk', *Health, Risk & Society* 16(1): 68–83.

Child, K. 2015. 'High Insurance Costs Scaring off Specialists'. Retrieved 17 June 2019 from http://www.timeslive.co.za/thetimes/2015/01/11/High-insurance-costs-scaring-off-specialists.

Clarke, A. 1995. 'Modernity, Postmodernity and Reproductive Processes ca. 1890-1990, or, Mommy, Where Do Cyborgs Come from Anyway?', in C. Gray, H. Figueroa-Serriera and S. Mentor (eds), *The Cyborg Handbook*. New York: Routledge.

Clarke, A., J. Shim, L. Mamo, J. Fosket and J. Fisherman. 2003. 'Biomedicalisation: Technoscientific Transformations of Health, Illness and US Biomedicine', *American Sociological Review* 68: 161–94.

Clarke, S. 1981. *The Foundations of Structuralism: A Critique of Claude Levi-Strauss and the Structuralist Movement*. Brighton: The Harvester Press Limited.

Clifford, J. and G. Marcus. 1986. *Writing Culture: The Poetics and Politics of Ethnography*. California: University of California Press.

Cock, J. 1980. *Maids and Madams*. Johannesburg: Raven Press.

Comaroff, J. 1985. *Body of Power, Spirit of Resistance: The Culture and History of a South African People*. Chicago: Chicago University Press.

Cosslett, T. 1994. *Women Writing Childbirth: Modern Discourses of Motherhood*. Manchester: Manchester University Press.

Crawshaw, P. 2012. 'Governing at a Distance: Social Marketing and the (Bio)politics of Responsibility', *Social Science and Medicine* 75(1): 200–207.

Csordas, T. 2002. *Body/Meaning/Healing*. New York: Palgrave Macmillan.

_____. 1994. *Embodiment and Experience: The Existential Ground of Culture and Self*. Cambridge: Cambridge University Press.

Daly, M. and J. Lewis. 2000. 'The Concept of Social Care and the Analysis of Contemporary Welfare States', *The British Journal of Sociology* 51(2): 281–98.

Das, V. 1996. 'Language and Body: Transactions in the Construction of Pain', *Daedalus* 125(1): 67–91.

_____. 2000. *Violence and Subjectivity*. California: University of California Press.

_____. 2007. *Life and Words: Violence and the Descent into the Ordinary*. Berkeley: University of California Press.

_____. 2010. 'Engaging the Life of the Other: Love and Everyday Life', in M. Lambek (ed.), *Ordinary Ethics*. New York: Fordham University Press.

Davis-Floyd, R. 1992. *Birth as an American Rite of Passage*. Berkeley: University of California Press.

_____. 1994. 'The Technocratic Body: American Childbirth as Cultural Expression', *Social Science and Medicine* 38(8): 1125–40.

Davis-Floyd, R. and C. Sargent (eds). 1997. *Childbirth and Authoritative Knowledge: Cross-cultural Perspectives*. Berkeley: University of California Press.

Deacon, H. 1998. 'Midwives and Medical Men in the Cape Colony before 1860', *The Journal of African History* 39(2): 271–92.

Deleuze, G. and F. Guattari. 1972. *Anti-Oedipus: Capitalism and Schizophrenia.* London: Penguin.

DeLoache, J. and A. Gottlieb. 2000. *A World of Babies: Imagined Childcare Guides for Seven Societies.* Cambridge: Cambridge University Press.

Devisch, R. 1985. 'Approaches to Symbol and Symptom in Bodily Space-time', *International Journal of Psychology* 20: 389–415.

Diamond, I. and L. Quinby. 1988. 'American Feminism and the Language of Control', in *Feminism and Foucault.* Boston, MA: Northeastern University Press.

Dick-Read, G. 1933. *Natural Childbirth.* London: Heinemann.

Digby, A. and H. Sweet. 2005. 'Race, Identity and the Nursing Profession: The 1949 Revolt of the African Nurse in South Africa', in S. McGann and B. Mortimer (eds), *New Directions in the History of Nursing: International Perspectives.* London: Routledge.

Dougherty, M. 1978. 'Southern Lay Midwives as Ritual Specialists', in J. Hoch-Smith and A. Spring (eds), *Women in Ritual and Symbolic Roles.* New York: Plenam.

Douglas, M. 1966. *Purity and Danger: An Analysis of Concepts of Pollution and Taboo.* London: Routledge and Kegan Paul.

_____. 1992. *Risk and Blame: Essays in Cultural Theory.* London: Routledge.

Douglas, M. and A. Wildavsky. 1982. *Risk and Culture: An Essay on the Selection of Technological and Environmental Dangers.* Los Angeles: University of California Press.

Dye, N. 1986. 'The Medicalisation of Birth', in P. Eakins (ed.), *The American Way of Birth.* Philadelphia, PA: Temple University Press.

Eisenstein, Z. 1988. *The Female Body and the Law.* Berkeley: University of California Press.

Evans, K. 2010. 'Independent Midwifery Practices in Cape Town: Birth Outcomes and Predictors for Medical Interventions from 2003–2009'. Unpublished Masters Dissertation, University of Cape Town.

Faircloth, C. 2009. 'Mothering as Identity-work: Long-term Breastfeeding and Intensive Motherhood', *Anthropology News* 2: 15–17.

Farmer, P. 1988. 'Bad Blood, Spoiled Milk: Bodily Fluids as Moral Barometers in Rural Haiti', *American Ethnologist* 15(1): 62–83.

_____. 1992. *Aids and Accusation: Haiti and the Geography of Blame.* Berkeley: University of California Press.

_____. 1996. 'Pathologies of Power: Rethinking Health and Human Rights', *American Journal of Public Health* 89(10): 1486–96.

_____. 1999. 'On Suffering and Violence: a View from Below', *Daedalus* 125(1): 261–83.

Farquhar, J. 2012. *Ten Thousand Things: Nurturing Life in Contemporary Beijing.* Brooklyn: Zone Books.

Farquhar, J. and M. Lock. 2007. *Beyond the Body Proper: Reading the Anthropology of Material Life.* Durham, NC: Duke University Press.

Farrell Krell, D. 2003. 'Far from the Pallid Float', in E. Hooke and W. Fuchs (eds), *Encounters with Alphonso Lingis.* Lanham, MD: Lexington Books.

Fassin, D. 2001. 'The Biopolitics of Otherness: Undocumented Foreigners and Racial Discrimination in French Public Debate', *Anthropology Today* 17(1): 3–7.

Fassin, D. and H. Schneider. 2003. 'The Politics of Aids in South Africa: Beyond the Controversies', *British Medical Journal* 326: 495–97.

Faubian, J. 2001. *The Ethics of Kinship.* Lanham, MD: Rowan and Littlefield Publishers.

Featherstone, M. 1991. 'The Body in Consumer Culture', in M. Featherstone, M. Hepworth and B. Turner (eds), *The Bbody: Social Process and Cultural Theory.* London: Sage.

Feder Kittay, E. and Diana T. Meyers. 1987. *Women and Moral Theory.* New Jersey: Rowman and Littlefield.

Feld, S., A. Fox, T. Porcello and D. Samuels. 2004. 'Vocal Anthropology: From the Music of Language to the Language of Song', in A. Duranti (ed.), *A Companion to Linguistic Anthropology.* Malden, MA: Blackwell.

Fenwick, J., L. Staff, J. Gamble, D. Creedy and S. Bayes. 2010. 'Why do Women Request Caesarean Section in a Normal, Healthy First Pregnancy?', *Midwifery* 26(4): 394–400.

Ferreira, N. 2016. 'Enduring "Lateness": Biomedicalisation and the Unfolding of

Reproductive Life, Sociality, and Antenatal Care'. Unpublished Masters thesis. University of Cape Town.

Finkler, K. 2003. 'Illusions of Controlling the Future: Risk and Genetic Inheritance', *Anthropology and Medicine* 10(1): 51–70.

Fisher, B. and J. Tronto. 1990. 'Towards a Feminist Theory of Caring', in E. Abel and M. Nelson (eds), *Circle of Care: Work and Identity in Women's Lives.* New York: SUNY Press.

Fisher, C., Y. Hauck and J. Fenwick. 2006. 'How Social Context Impacts on Women's Fears of Childbirth: A Western Australian Example', *Social Science and Medicine* 63(1): 64–75.

Fokazi, S. 2011. 'Experts Call for Cut in C-section Birth Rates'. Retrieved 10 June 2016 from https://www.iol.co.za/lifestyle/family/pregnancy/experts-call-for-cut-in-c-section-birth-rates-1029667.

Fonn, S., M. Xaba, K. Tint, D. Conco and S. Varkey. 1998. 'Maternal Health Services in South Africa', *South African Medical Journal* 88: 697–702.

Foreman, A. 1977. *Femininity as Alienation.* London: Pluto Press.

Foucault, M. 1977. *Discipline and Punish: The Birth of the Prison.* Trans. A. Sheridan. New York: Pantheon Books.

_____. 1986. *The History of Sexuality, vol. 3. The Care of the Self.* New York: Vintage.

Franklin, S. 1997. *Embodied Progress: A Cultural Account of Assisted Conception.* London: Routledge.

Franklin, S. and S. McKinnon. 2001. *Relative Values: Reconfiguring Kinship Study.* Durham, NC: Duke University Press.

Fraser, G. 1992. *Afro-American Midwives, Biomedicine and the State.* Cambridge: Harvard University Press.

Fraser, N. 1997. 'Heterosexism, Misrecognition and Capitalism: A Response to Judith Butler', *Social Text* 52/53: 279–89.

Garcia, A. 2010. *The Pastoral Clinic: Addiction and Dispossession along the Rio Grande.* Berkeley: University of California Press.

Geertz, C. 1974. 'From the Native's Point of View: on the Nature of Anthropological Understanding'. Reprinted in 1984 in R. Shweder and R. LeVine (eds), *Culture Theory.* Cambridge: Cambridge University Press.

Giddens, A. and J. Turner. 1987. *Social Theory Today.* Stanford, CA: Stanford University Press.

Gilligan, C. 1982. *In a Different Voice: Psychological Theory and Women's Development.* Cambridge: Harvard University Press.

Ginsburg, F. 1987. 'Procreation Stories: Reproduction, Nurturance and Procreation in Life Narratives of Abortion Activists', *American Ethnologist* 14(4): 623–36.

Ginsburg, F. and R. Rapp. 1991. 'The Politics of Reproduction', *Annual Review of Anthropology* 20: 311–43.

Ginsburg, F. and R. Rapp. 1995. *Conceiving the New World Order: The Global Politics of Reproduction.* Berkeley: University of California Press.

Glenn, E. 1994. 'Social Constructions of Mothering: a Thematic Overview', in E. Glenn and G. Chang (eds), *Mothering: Ideology, Experience and Agency.* New York: Routledge.

Goffman, E. 1957. 'Alienation from Interaction', *Human Relations* 10(1): 47–60.

Good, B. and M.J. DelVecchio Good. 1993. '"Learning Medicine": The Constructing of Medical Knowledge at Harvard Medical School', in S. Lindenbaum and M. Lock (eds), *Knowledge, Power and Practice: The Anthropology of Medicine and Everyday Life.* Berkeley: University of California Press.

Gray, A., Y. Vawda and C. Jack. 2013. 'Health Policy and Legislation', in *South African Health Review.* Durban: Health Systems Trust.

Greenlees, J. 2015. *Western Modernity and Medicine 1880–1990.* New York: Routledge.

Greenspan, M. 1983. *A New Approach to Women and Therapy.* New York: McGraw-Hill.

Grosz, E. 1994. *Volatile Bodies: Toward a Corporeal Feminism.* Bloomington: Indiana University Press.

_____. 2003. 'Naked', in E. Hooke and W. Fuchs (eds), *Encounters with Alphonso Lingis.* Lanham, MD: Lexington Books.

Hacking, I. 1996. 'Normal People', in D. Olsen and N. Torrance (eds), *Modes of Thought.* Cambridge: Cambridge University Press.

Han, C. 2012. *Life in Debt: Times of Care and Violence in Neoliberal Chile.* Berkeley: University of California Press.

Han, S. 2013. *Pregnancy in Practice: Expedition and Experience in the Contemporary US.* New York: Berghahn Books.

Hanson, C. 2004. *A Cultural History of Pregnancy: Pregnancy, Medicine and Culture, 1750–2000.* Hampshire: Palgrave Macmillan.

Havel, V. 1983. *Letters to Olga.* New York: Holt.

Held, V. 1993. *Feminist Morality: Transforming Culture, Society and Politics.* Chicago: University of Chicago Press.

Hellman, C. 2000. *Culture, Health and Illness.* London: Butterworth-Heinemann.

Henderson, P. 2012. *A Kinship of Bones: AIDS, Intimacy and Care in Rural Kwazulu-Natal.* Durban: UKZN Press.

Hills-Collins, P. 1991. *Black Feminist Thought: Knowledge, Consciousness and the Power of Empowerment.* New York: Routledge.

Hofmeyr, G., V. Nikodem, W. Wolman, B. Chalmers and T. Kramer. 1991. 'Companionship to Modify the Clinical Birth Environment: Effects on Progress and Perceptions of Labour, and Breastfeeding', *British Journal of Obstetrics and Gynaecology* 98: 756–64.

Howell, S. 2003. 'Kinning: The Creation of Life Trajectories in Transnational Adoptive Families', *Journal of the Royal Anthropological Institute* 9: 465–84.

Hugh-Jones, C. 1979. *From the Milk River: Spatial and Temporal Processes in North-west Amazonia.* Cambridge: Cambridge University Press.

Humphreys, K. 1998. 'Medicalised Maternity: an Investigation into Women's Experiences of Medicalised Childbirth'. Unpublished Masters thesis. Cape Town: University of Cape Town.

Hunt, L., H. Casteneda and K. DeVoogd. 2006. 'Do Notions of Risk Inform Patient Choice? Lessons from a Study of Prenatal Genetic Counselling', *Medical Anthropology* 25(3): 193–219.

Hunter, C. 2012. Intimate Space within Institutionalised Birth: Women's Experiences Birthing with Doulas', *Anthropology and Medicine* 19(3): 315–26.

Ingold, T. 2000. *The Perception of the Environment: Essays on Livelihood, Dwelling Skill.* New York: Routledge.

Irigaray, L. 1993. *An Ethics of Sexual Difference.* Ithaca, NY: Cornell University Press.

Jewkes, R., N. Abrahams and Z. Mvo. 1998. 'Why do Nurses Abuse Patients? Reflections from South African Obstetric Services', *Social Science and Medicine* 47: 1781–95.

Jordan, B. 1978. *Birth in Four Cultures: A Crosscultural Investigation of Childbirth in Yucatan, Holland, Sweden and the United States.* Montreal: Eden Press.

Katzenellenbogen, J. and R. Dorrington. 1993. 'Mortality in a Rural South African Mission, 1837–1909: An Historical Cohort Study using Church Records', *International Journal of Epidemiology* 22: 965–75.

Katz-Rothman, B. 1982. *In Labour: Women and Power in the Birthplace.* New York: W.W. Norton and Co. Inc.

Kaufman, S. 2005. *...And a Time to Die: How American Hospitals Shape the End of Life*. Chicago: University of Chicago Press.

Kelly, T. 2013. 'A Life Less Miserable?', *HAU: Journal of Ethnographic Theory* 3(1): 213–16.

Kitzinger, S. 1962/1981. *The Experience of Childbirth*. London: Penguin.

_____. 1992. 'Birth and Violence against Women: Generating Hypotheses from Women's Accounts of Unhappiness after Childbirth', in H. Roberts (ed.), *Women's Health Matters*. New York Psychology Press.

_____. 2002. 'What Do We Tell the Children?' *Birth: Issues in Perinatal Care* 29(1): 60–61.

_____. 2005. *The Politics of Birth*. Edinburgh: Elsevier.

Klassen, P. 2001. 'Maternities and Postbiomedical Bodies: Religion and Nature in Contemporary Homebirth', *Signs* 26(3): 775–809.

Klein, J. 2016. 'Get the Epidural'. Retrieved 17 June 2019 from http://www.nytimes.com/2016/07/10/opinion/sunday/get-the-epidural.html.

Kleinman, A. 1988. 'The Illness Narratives: Suffering, Healing and the Human Condition'. New York: Basic Books.

_____. 2009. 'Caregiving: The Odyssey of Becoming More Human', *The Lancet* 373 (9660): 292–293.

_____. 2015. 'The Art of Medicine: Care, in Search of a Health Agenda', *The Lancet* 386(9990): 240–241.

Kleinman, A. and J. Kleinman. 1994. 'How Bodies Remember: Social Memory and Bodily Experience of Criticism, Resistance and Delegitimation Following China's Cultural Revolution'. *New Literary History* 25(3): 707–723.

Kobrin, F. 1966. 'The American Midwife Controversy', *Bulletin of the History of Medicine* 40(4): 350–363.

Kopas, L. 2014. 'A Review of Evidence Based Practices for Management of the Second Stage of Labour'. *Journal of Midwifery and Women's Health* 59(3): 264–276.

Kristeva, J. 1985. 'Stabat Mater', *Poetics Today* 6(1/2): 133–152.

Kruger, L.-M. 2003. 'Narrating Motherhood: The Transformative Potential of Individual Stories', *South African Journal of Psychology* 33(4): 198–204.

Labov, W. 1984. 'Intensity', in D. Schiffren (ed.), *Meaning, Form and Use in Context: Linguistic Applications, GURT '84*. Washington: Georgetown University Press.

Laderman, C. 1983. 'Wives and Midwives: Childbirth and Nutrition in Rural Malaysia'. Berkeley: University of California Press.

_____. 1994. 'The Embodiment of Symbols and the Acculturation of the Anthropologist', in T. Csordas (ed.), *Embodiment and Experience: The Existential Ground of Culture and Self*. Cambridge: Cambridge University Press.

Laidlaw, J. 1995. *Riches and Renunciation: Religion, Economy and Society among the Jains*. Oxford: Oxford University Press.

Lakoff, G. and M. Johnson. 1980. *Metaphors We Live By*. Chicago: Chicago University Press.

Lalor, J.D. Devane and C. Begley. 2007. 'Unexpected Diagnosis of Foetal Abnormality: Women's Encounters with Caregivers', *Birth* 34(1): 80–88.

Lambek, M. 1998. *Bodies and Persons: Comparative Perspectives from Africa and Melanesia*. Cambridge: Cambridge University Press.

Lambert, H. 1992. 'The Cultural Logic of Indian Medicine: Prognosis and Etiology in Rajashthani Popular Therapeutics', *Social Science and Medicine* 34(10): 1069–76.

Lapperman, M. 2011. 'The Exploration of Elective Caesarean Sections as a Choice Around Childbirth'. Unpublished MA dissertation, University of Cape Town.

Latour, Bruno. 2007. 'The Recall of Modernity', *Cultural Studies Review* 13(1): 11–30.

Lavender, T., E. Campbell, S. Thompson and L. Briscoe. 2003. 'Supplying Women with Evidence-based Information', *Foundation of Nursing Studies Dissemination Series: Developing Practice Improving Care* 2(4): 1–4.

Leavitt, J. 1986. *Brought to Bed: Child-bearing in America, 1750–1950*. New York: Oxford University Press.

Lefebvre, H. 2004. *Rhythmanalysis: Space, Time and Everyday Life*. London: Continuum.

Levi-Strauss, C. 1963. *Structural Anthropology*. New York: Basic Books.

_____. 1978. *Myth and Meaning*. Toronto: University of Toronto Press.

Lindmeier, C. 2015. 'Caesarean Sections Should Only Be Performed when Medically Necessary'. Retrieved 10 May 2019 from https://www.who.int/mediacentre/news/releases/2015/caesarean-sections/en/.

Lingis, A. 1994. *The Community of Those Who Have Nothing in Common*. Bloomington: Indiana University Press.

_____. 2003. 'Trust', in E. Hooke and W. Fuchs (eds), *Encounters with Alphonso Lingis*. Lanham, MD: Lexington Books.

_____. 2004. *Trust*. Minneapolis: University of Minnesota Press.

Lippi-Green, R. 2012. *English with an Accent: Language, Ideology and Discrimination in the United States*. New York: Routledge.

Livingston, J. 2012. *Improvising Medicine: An African Oncology Ward in an Emerging Cancer Epidemic*. Durham, NC: Duke University Press.

Lock, M. 1991. 'Contesting Meanings of the Menopause', *Lancet* 337: 1270–91.

_____. 1993. 'Cultivating the Body: Anthropology and Epistemologies of Bodily Practice and Knowledge', *Annual Review of Anthropology* 22: 133–55.

Lock, M. and P. Kaufert (eds). 1998. *Pragmatic Women and Body Politics*. Cambridge: Cambridge University Press.

Lock, M. and V.K. Nguyen. 2010. *An Anthropology of Biomedicine*. Chichester: John Wiley and Sons.

Lock, M. and N. Scheper-Hughes. 1987. 'The Mindful Body: A Prolegomenon to Future Work in Medical Anthropology'. *Medical Anthropology Quarterly* 1(1): 6–41.

Lowe, N. 2002. 'The Nature of Labour Pain', *American Journal of Obstetrics and Gynaecology* 186(5): 16–24.

Lupton, D. 1999. *Risk and Sociocultural Theory: New Directions and Perspectives.* Cambridge: Cambridge University Press.

MacCormack, C. 1982. *Ethnography of Fertility and Birth.* New York: Academic Press.

MacDonald, M. 2008. *At Work in the Field of Birth: Midwifery Narratives of Nature, Tradition and Home.* Nashville: Vanderbilt University Press.

Maclean, L., M. McDermott and C. May. 2000. 'Method of Delivery and Subjective Distress: Women's Emotional Responses to Childbirth Practices', *Journal of Reproductive and Infant Psychology* 18(2): 153–62.

Macleod, C. and K. Durrheim. 2002. 'Racialising Teenage Pregnancy: "Culture" and "Tradition" in the South African Scientific Literature'. Unpublished manuscript.

Maher, J. 2008. 'Progressing through Labour and Delivery: Birth Time and Women's Experiences', *Women's Studies International Forum* 31(2): 129–37.

Malinowski, B. 1962. *Sex, Culture and Myth.* New York: Harcourt, Brace and World.

Marks, S. 1994. *Divided Sisterhood: Race, Class and Gender in the South African Nursing Profession.* London: Palgrave Macmillan.

Marriot, M. 1976. 'Hindu Transactions', in B. Kapferer (ed.), *Transaction and Meaning: Directions in the Anthropology of Exchange and Symbolic Behaviour.* Philadelphia: Inst. Study Human Issues.

Martin, E. 1987. *The Woman in the Body: A Cultural Analysis of Reproduction.* Boston, MA: Beacon Press.

_____. 1997. 'The End of the Body?', in R. Lancaster and M. di Leonardo (eds), *The Gender Sexuality Reader.* New York: Routledge.

Mattingly, C. 1998. 'In Search of the Good: Narrative Reasoning in Clinical Practice', *Medical Anthropology Quarterly* 12(3): 273–97.

Mauss, M. 1935. 'Techniques of the Body', *Economy and Society* 2: 70–88.

_____. 1954. *The Gift: Forms and Functions of Exchange in Archaic Societies.* London: Cohen and West.

May, J. (ed.) 2000. *Poverty and Inequality in South Africa.* Cape Town: David Philip.

Mayeroff, M. 1971. *On Caring.* New York: Harper Collins.

McCabe, K. 2016. 'Mothercraft: Birth Work and the Making of Neoliberal Mothers', *Social Science and Medicine* 162: 177–84.

McClain, C. 1975. 'Ethno-obstetrics in Ajijic', *Anthropological Quarterly* 48(1): 38–56.

McPherson, N. 2011. 'Afterward', in N. McPherson and M. Walks (eds), *An Anthropology of Mothering.* Bradford: Demeter Press.

Millennium Development Goals (MGD). 2000. UN General Assembly, United Nations Millennium Declaration, Resolution Adopted by the

General Assembly, 18 September 2000, A/RES/55/2. Retrieved 2 July 2019 from https://www.refworld.org/docid/3b00f4ea3.html.

Melzack, R., P. Taenzer, P. Feldman and R. Kinch. 1981. 'Labour is Still Painful after Prepared Childbirth Training', *CMA Journal* 24: 357–63.

Merleau-Ponty, M. 1962. *Phenomenology of Perception.* London: Routledge and Kegan Paul Ltd.

Mol, A. 2002. *The Body Multiple: Ontology in Medical Practice.* Durham, NC: Duke University Press.

_____. 2008. *The Logic of Care: Health and Problem of Patient Choice.* New York: Routledge.

Mongan, M. 1992. *Hypnobirthing: The Mongan Method.* Florida: Health Communications.

Morgan, L. 2009. *Icons of Life: A Cultural History of Human Embryos.* Berkeley: University of California Press.

Mulkay, M.J. and G. Nigel Gilbert. 1982. 'What is the Ultimate Question?', *Social Studies of Science* 12: 309–19.

Murphy, E. 1999. '"Breast is Best": Infant Feeding Decisions and Maternal Deviance', *Sociology of Health and Illness* 21(2): 187–208.

Nader, L. 1969. 'Up the Anthropologist: Perspectives Gained from Studying up', in D. Hymes (ed.), *Reinventing Anthropology.* New York: Random House.

Narayan, K. 1993. 'How Native Is the "Native" Anthropologist?' *American Anthropologist* 95(3): 671–686.

Nash, M. 2012. *Making Postmodern Mothers: Pregnant Embodiment, Baby Bumps and Body Image.* Basingstoke: Palgrave MacMillan.

Newman, K. 1996. *Foetal Positions: Individualism, Science and Visuality*. Stanford: Stanford University Press.

Newman, L. 1981. 'Midwives and Modernisation', *Medical Anthropology* 5(1): 1–12.

Newton, B., J. Southall, J. Raphael, R. Ashford and K. LeMarchand. 2002. 'A Narrative Review of the Impact of Disbelief in Chronic Pain', *Pain Management Nursing* 14(3): 161–71.

Ngubane, H. 1977. *Body and Mind in Zulu Medicine.* New York: Academic.

Nichter, M. 2003. 'Harm Reduction: A Core Concern for Medical Anthropology', in B. Harthorn and L. Oaks (eds), *Risk, Culture and Health Inequality: Shifting Perceptions of Danger and Blame.* Westport: Greenwood Publishing Group.

Noddings, N. 1984. *Caring: A Feminine Approach to Ethics and Moral Education.* Berkeley: University of California Press.

Nussbaum, M. 2005. 'Women's Bodies: Violence, Security and Capabilities', *Journal of Human Development* 6(2): 167–83.

Nyamnjoh, F. 2015. 'Beyond and Evangelising Public Anthropology: Science, Theory and Commitment', *Journal of Contemporary African Studies* 33(1): 48–63.

O'Neil, J. and P. Kaufert. 1990. 'Cooptation and Control: The Reconstruction of Innuit Birth', *Medical Anthropology Quarterly* 4(4): 427–42.

Oakley, A. 1979. *Becoming a Mother.* New York: Schocken.

_____. 1980. *Women Confined: Towards a Sociology of Childbirth.* Oxford: Martin Robertson.

Ochs, E. and L. Capps. 1996. 'Narrating the Self', *Annual Review of Anthropology* 25: 19–43.

Odent, M. 1984. *Birth Reborn: What Childbirth Should Be.* New York: Pantheon.

Ong, A. 1995. 'Women out of China: Travelling Tales and Travelling Theories in Postcolonial Feminism', in R. Behar and D. Gordon (eds), *Women Writing Culture.* Berkeley: University of California Press.

Ortner, S. 1972. 'Is Female to Male as Nature is to Culture', *Feminist Studies* 1(2): 5–31.

Packard, R. 1996. 'Review: A History of Nursing'. *The Journal of African History* 37(2): 324–326.

Parish, S. 1991. 'The Sacred Mind: Newar Cultural Representations of Mental Life and the Production of Moral Consciousness', *Ethos* 19(3): 313–51.

Parsons, T. 1964. *Social Structure and Personality.* New York: The Free Press of Glencoe.

Paxson, H. 2004. *Making Modern Mothers: Ethics and Family Planning in Rrban Greece.* Berkeley: University of California Press.

_____. 2002. 'Rationalising Sex: Family Planning and the Making of Modern Mothers in Urban Greece', *American Ethnologist* 29(2): 307–34.

Penn-Kekana, L. and D. Blaauw. 2002. 'A Rapid Appraisal of Maternal Health Services in South Africa: A Health Systems Approach'. Johannesburg: The Centre for Health Policy School of Public Health, University of the Witswatersrand.

Penn-Kekana, L., B. McPake and J. Parkhurst. 2007. 'Improving Maternal Health: Getting What Works to Happen'. *Reproductive Health Matters* 15(30): 28–37.

Petchesky, R. 1995. 'The Body as Property: A Feminist Re-vision', in F. Ginsburg and R. Rapp (eds), *Conceiving the New World Order: The Global Politics of Reproduction.* Berkeley: University of California Press.

Pillay, R. 2009. 'Work Satisfaction of Professional Nurses in South Africa: A Comparative Analysis of the Private and Public Sectors', *Human Resources for Health* 7(15).

Popke, J. 2006. 'Geography and Ethics: Everyday Mediations Through Care and Consumption', *Progress in Human Geography* 30(4): 504–12.

Povinelli, E. 2002. *The Cunning of Recognition: Indigenous Alterities and the Making of Australian Multiculturalism.* Durham, NC: Duke University Press.

Radley, A. 1994. *Making Sense of Illness: The Social Psychology of Pain and Disease.* Thousand Oaks,CA: Sage.

Rahaim, M. 2012. *Musicking Bodies: Gesture and Voice in Hindustani Music.* Middletown: Wesleyan University Press.

Rapp, R. 1989. 'Chromosomes and Communication: The Discourse of Genetic Counseling', in L. Whiteford and M. Poland (eds), *New Approaches to Human Reproduction: Social and Ethical Dimensions.* Boulder, CO: Westview Press.

_____. 1993. 'Amniocentesis in Sociocultural Perspective', *Journal of Genetic Counselling* 2(4): 183–96.

_____. 1999. *Testing Women, Testing the Foetus: The Social Impact of Amniocentesis in America.* New York: Routledge.

Reddy, V., S. Meyer, T. Shefer and T. Meyiwe (eds). 2014. *Care in Context: Transnational Gender Perspectives.* South Africa: HSRC Press.

Reed, R. 2013. *Midwifery Practice during Childbirth: Rites of Passage and Rites of Protection.* Unpublished PhD dissertation, University of the Sunshine Coast.

Reid, M. 1989. 'Sisterhood and Professionalism: A Case Study of the American Lay Midwife', in C. McClain (ed.), *Women as Healers: Cross-cultural Perspectives.* New Brunswick: Rutgers University Press.

Rich, A. 1976. *Of Woman Born: Motherhood as Experience and Institution.* New York: W.W. Norton and Company.

Richardson, J. 2005. 'Establishing the (Extra)ordinary in Chronic Widespread Pain', *Health* 9(1): 31–48.

Ricoeur, P. 1981. 'Narrative Time', in W. Mitchell (ed.), *On Narrative.* Chicago: Chicago University Press.

Robbins, J. 2013. 'Beyond the Suffering Subject: Toward an Anthropology of the Good', *Journal of the Royal Anthropological Institute* 19(3): 447–62.

Robinson, F. 1999. *Globalising Care: Ethics, Feminist Theory and International Relations.* Boulder, CO: Westview Press.

Ross. F. 2010. *Raw Life, New Hope: Decency, Housing and Everyday Life in a Post-apartheid Community.* Cape Town: UCT Press.

_____. 2014. 'Mother of Two Children', *Anthropology Southern Africa* 37(1 and 2): 50–61.

Rothman, B. 1983. Midwives in Transition: The Structure of a Clinical Revolution, *Social Problems* 30(3): 262–271.

Roux, S. and L. van Rensburg. 2011. South African Mothers' Perceptions and Experiences of Unplanned Caesarean Sections, *Journal of Psychology in Africa* 21(3): 429–438.

Ruddick, S. 1980. *Maternal Thinking*, Boston: Beacon Press.

South African Health Review (SAHR) 2012/2013. 2013. Ed. A. Padarath and R. English. Cape Town: Health Systems Trust.

Sargent, C. 1989. *Maternity, Medicine and Power: Reproductive Decisions in Urban Benin.* Berkeley: University of California Press.

Scarry, E. 1985. *The Body in Pain: The Making and Unmaking of the World.* Oxford: Oxford University Press.

Scheper-Hughes, N. (ed.). 1987. *Child Survival: Anthropological Perspectives on the Treatment and Maltreatment of Children.* Dordrecht: Reidel.

Searle, C. 1965. *The History of the Development of Nursing in South Africa 1652–1960*. Cape Town: Struik.

Sevenhuijsen, S. 1998. *Citizenship and the Ethics of Care: Feminist Considerations on Justice, Morality and Politics*. London: Routledge.

_____. 2000. 'Caring in the Third Way: The Relation Between Obligation, Responsibility and Care in Third Way Discourse', *Critical Social Policy* 20(1): 5–37.

_____. 2003. 'South African Social Welfare Policy: An Approach through the Ethic of Care', *Critical Social Policy* 23(3): 299–321.

Shaw, N. 1974. *Forced Labour: Maternity Care in the US*. New York: Pergamon Press.

Shaw, R. 2002. 'The Ethics of the Birth Plan in Childbirth Management Practices', *Feminist Theory* 3(2): 131–49.

Sidnell, J. 2010. 'The Ordinary Ethics of Everyday Talk', in M. Lambek (ed.), *Ordinary Ethics*. New York: Fordham University Press.

Smith, D. 2014. 'Caesarean Sections in South Africa "Recklessly High", Warn Experts'. Retrieved 17 June 2019 from https://www.theguardian.com/world/2014/sep/24/caesarean-section-south-africa.

Sobo, E. 1995. *Choosing Unsafe Sex: Aids-risk Denial among Disadvantaged Women*. Philadelphia: University of Pennsylvania Press.

Song, F., J. West, L. Lundy and N. Dahmen. 2012. 'Women, Pregnancy, and Health Information Online: The Making of Informed Patients and Ideal Mothers', *Gender & Society* 26(5): 773–98.

Sontag, S. 1978. *Illness as Metaphor*. New York: Farrar, Straus and Giroux.

Spelman, E. 1982. 'Women as Body: Ancient and Contemporary Views', *Feminist Studies* 8(1): 109–31.

Strathern, M. 1984. 'Subject or Object? Women and the Circulation of Valuables in Highlands New Guinea', in R. Hirschon (ed.), *Women and Property, Women as Property*. New York: St. Martin's Press.

_____. 1988. 'Anthropological Strategies', and 'Cause and Effect', in *The Gender of the Gift*. Cambridge: Cambridge University Press.

_____. 1995. 'Displacing Knowledge: Technology and the Consequences for Kinship', in F. Ginsburg and R. Rapp (eds), *Conceiving the New World Order: The Global Politics of Reproduction*. Berkeley: University of California Press.

Taussig, K. 2009. *Ordinary Genomes: Science, Citizenship and Genetic Identities (Experimental Futures)*. Durham, NC: Duke University Press.

Taylor, J. 2000. 'Of Sonograms and Baby Prams: Prenatal Diagnosis, Pregnancy, and Consumption', *Feminist Studies* 25(2): 391–418.

Ticktin, M. 2011. *Casualties of Care: Immigration and the Politics of Humanitarianism in France*. Berkeley: University of California Press.

Tieks, F., A. Lam and B. Matta. 1995. 'Effects of Valsalva Manoeuvre on Cerebral Circulation in Healthy Adults: A Transcranial Doppler Study'. *Stroke* 26(8): 1386–1392.

Tlebere, P., D. Jackson, M. Loveday, L. Matizirofa, N. Mbombo, T. Doherty, A. Wigton, L. Treger and M. Chopra. 2007. 'Community Based Situation

Analysis of Maternal and Neonatal Care in South Africa to Explore Factors that Impact Utilization of Maternal Health Services', *Journal of Midwifery and Women's Health* 52: 342–50.

Treichler, P. 1990. 'Feminism, Medicine and Meaning of Childbirth', in M. Jocobus, E. Keller and S. Shuttleworth. *Body/Politic, Women and the Discourse of Science*. New York and London: Routledge.

Tshwane Declaration of support for breastfeeding. 2011. *South African Journal of Nutrition* 24(4): 214.

Torres, J. 2015. 'Families, Markets and Medicalisation: The Role of Paid Support for Childbirth and Breastfeeding', *Qualitative Health Research* 25(7): 899–911.

Tronto, J. 1989. 'Women and Caring: Or, What Can Feminists Learn From Caring?', in A. Jaggar and S. Bordo (eds), *Gender/Body/Knowledge Feminist Reconstructions of Being and Knowing*. New Brunswick: Rutgers University Press.

_____. 1993. *Moral Boundaries: A Political Argument for an Ethic of Care*. New York: Routledge.

_____. 2005. 'An Ethic of Care', A. Cudd and R. Andreasen (eds), *Feminist Theory: A Philosophical Anthology*. Malden: Blackwell Publishing.

_____. 2006. 'Gender, Ethics and Political Theory', in K. Davis, M. Evans and J. Lorber (eds), *Handbook of Gender and Women's Studies*. Thousand Oaks, CA: Sage.

_____. 2010. 'Creating Caring Institutions: Politics, Plurality, and Purpose', *Ethics and Social Welfare* 4(2): 158–71.

Tully, K. and H. Ball. 2013. 'Misrecognition of Need: Women's Experiences of and Explanations for Undergoing Caesarean Delivery', *Social Science and Medicine* 85: 103–11.

Turner, T. 1980. 'The Social Skin', in J. Cherfas and R. Lewin (eds), *Not Work Alone*. London: Temple Smith.

_____. 1993. 'Anthropology and Multiculturalism: What is Anthropology that Multiculturalists should be Mindful of?', *Cultural Anthropology* 8(4): 411–29.

United Nations, General Assembly. 2000. Millennium declaration. 55th session. Agenda item 60 (b).

Van Gennep, A. 1906 (in French) and 1960. *The Rites of Passage*. Chicago: University of Chicago Press.

Van Hollen, C. 2003a. *Birth on the Threshold: Childbirth and Modernity in South India*. Berkeley: University of California Press.

_____. 2003b. 'Invoking Vali Painful Technologies of Modern Birth in South India', *Medical Anthropology Quarterly* 17(1): 49.

Visagie, J. and D. Posel. 2011. 'A Reconsideration of What and Who Is Middle-class in South Africa'. Working paper 249. University of Kwazulu Natal.

Vivian, L., C. Naidu, M. Keikelame and J. Irlam. 2011. 'Medical Students' Experiences of Professional Lapses and Patients' Rights Abuses in a South African Health Sciences Faculty', *Academic Medicine* 86: 10.
Waltz, M. 2014. 'Milk and Management: Breastfeeding as a Project', *Anthropology Southern Africa* 37(1 and 2): 42–49.
Weidman, A. 2014. 'Anthropology and Voice', *Annual Review of Anthropology* 43: 37–51.
Werner, A. and K. Malterud. 2003. 'It Is Hard Work Behaving as a Credible Patient: Encounters between Women with Chronic Pain and Their Doctors', *Social Science and Medicine* 57: 1409–19.
Wertz, D. and R. Wertz. 1977. *Lying in: A History of Childbirth in America*. New York: Free Press.
Wetherell, M. and J. Potter. 1992. *Mapping the Language of Racism: Discourse and the Legitimation of Exploitation*. New York: Columbia University Press.
White, J. 1999. 'Review: Citizenship and the Ethics of Care: Feminist Considerations on Justice, Morality and Politics', *Journal of Politics* 61(4): 1199–1201.
World Health Organisation (WHO). 2015. World Health Statistics 2015. WHO: Luxembourg.
World Health Organisation (WHO). 2017. World Health Statistics 2017. WHO: Luxembourg.
'Why South Africans Choose Caesars when Giving Birth'. 2014. http://www.timeslive.co.za/local/2014/09/22/why-south-africans-choose-caesars-when-giving-birth.
Williams, F. 2001. 'In and Beyond New Labour: Toward a New Political Ethic of Care', *Critical Social Policy* 21(4): 467–93.
The World Bank. 2015. 'Maternal Mortality Ratio (Modelled eEstimate, per 100 000 Live Births)'. Retrieved 10 May 2019 from https://data.worldbank.org/indicator/sh.sta.mmrt.
Xaba, W. 2017. 'Challenging Fanon: A Black Radical Feminist Perspective on Violence and the Fees Must Fall Movement', *Agenda* 31(3–4): 96–104.
Yildirim, G. and N. Beji. 2008. 'Effects of Pushing Techniques in Birth on Mother and Foetus: A Randomised Study' *Birth* 35(1): 25–30.
Young, I. 1979. 'Is There a Women's World? – Some Reflections of the Struggles for our Bodies', *Proceedings of 'the Second Sex – Thirty Years Later'. A Commemorative Conference on Feminist Theory*. New York: Humanities Institute.
_____. 1983. 'Rights to Intimacy in a Complex Society', *Journal of Social Philosophy* 14(2): 47–52.
_____. 1984. 'Pregnant Embodiment: Subjectivity and Alienation', *Journal of Medical Philosophy* 9(1): 45–62.
Yuval-Davis, N. 1999. 'Ethnicity, Gender Relations and Multiculturalism', in R. Torres, L. Miron and J. Inda (eds), *Race, Identity & Citizenship. A Reader*. Oxford: Blackwell.
Zigon, J. 2008. *Morality: An Anthropological Perspective*. Oxford: Berg Publishers.

Index

A
accompaniment, 6, 88, 94, 148–153
affect, 11, 21, 167–168
alienation, 62, 88, 90–91, 94–95, 144–145
attentiveness, 60, 88, 133–136, 152–154
Avishai, Orit, 56–60, 76, 88–89

B
binary, 17, 19, 26–27
birth, 36, 46–47, 73, 88–91
  as an experience, 105–106, 109–117, 123–124, 129–131, 133–134

C
Cape Town, 16, 104, 107
  history of, 28–29
  midwives, 12, 23, 36, 45, 61
  Southern suburbs, 16
capital, 27, 99, 125, 161
capitalism, 90
care, 12, 19–22
  care world, 9, 18, 108
  ethics of, 11–12, 23
  as a problem, 160–164
  theorising, 11
care work, 20, 76, 79–82, 87, 93, 133–134, 144–148, 152, 158–161
childbirth classes, 99
choice, 84, 91–94, 165
  ethics, 110–113
  informed, 151
  modernity, 65
  planning and knowing, 67
  responsiblisation, 125–130
  risk, 69–71
contractions, 104–105, 120, 169
control, 37–38, 48–49
colonial, 28–30, 59–62, 74–78
Cosslett, Tess, 26–30, 35

D
decision-making, 4, 34, 47, 59, 76–78, 89
depression, 17, 164
disempowerment, 46
doula, 8, 40, 112–113, 154

E
embodied, 15, 36, 60, 79, 89–91, 134, 141–143, 152, 158
embodiment, 36, 79, 115, 141
emotional work, 81, 84, 88–93, 152, 160–162
empowerment, 29, 66, 71, 91, 93, 99, 127–129
epidural, 5, 44, 49, 65–66, 95–98, 107–111, 113–115, 171

F
familiarity, 133, 136, 149–159

Farmer, Paul, 125
feminism, 33, 109, 127
Foucault, Michel, 155
Fraser, Nancy, 91–93

G
Ginsburg, Faye, 97–98, 126–129
Grosz, Elizabeth, 154
groundedness, 146–153

H
hypnobirthing, 120–124

I
identity, 79, 128
insider, 17, 20
international debates on birth, 7, 33
intervention, 25–28, 35, 40–48, 55,
  definition of, 21
  history, 28, 32
  note on, 18–20
intimacy, 134, 137, 153–158
limits of, 134, 137, 153–162
intuition, 36, 59, 81
isolation, 94–95, 129–131, 161

K
knowing, ways of, 38–39, 44, 59, 90
knowledge, 10, 29–31, 43, 84–87
  embodied, 36–38, 142–144
  lay, 11

L
language, 48, 79, 116, 130–131
  hypnobirthing, 105, 119–124
  metaphor, 99–102
  pain, 98, 111–115
  support, 73–74, 79, 80–81, 153, 168
  time, 18
Levi-Strauss, Claude, 27, 55–56, 123
Lingis, Alphonso, 151–152

M
medical system, 36
medicalisation, 8, 14, 28, 31, 33, 36
method, 13
middle-class, 3, 16–17, 20, 28, 49–51, 54–59, 67, 76, 92, 131, 161
midwives, 4–9
modern, 32, 59–60, 65, 89–91, 94–95, 129–131
modernity, 59, 79, 125,
motherhood, 26, 36, 58, 76, 88, 94, 98, 117, 125–131
myth, 42–43, 50, 54–57, 123

O
obstetrician, 6, 8, 15, 19, 26, 39, 41–44, 70–71, 93, 141
Odent, Michel, 51–52
outsider, 17, 20

P
pain, 97–102, 104–108
partner, 84, 140–145
planning, 58–65, 74, 76, 94–95
postnatal, 16–17, 121, 159–160
Povinelli, Elizabeth, 92–93, 165
pregnancy, as an experience, 67
preparation, 34, 50, 60–61, 101–102, 113, 118–119, 127–129
problem, care as a, 155, 160, 164–165
project, pregnancy as, 58–62

R
Rapp, Rayna, 15, 75
reassurance, 62, 84–88
recognition, 11–12, 71–72, 91–93, 130
relationality, 19, 154–155
responsiveness, 133–134, 146–149, 151–156
rights, 33, 53, 59, 72, 93
risk, 72–75, 78–82, 90–93, 95, 172–176

S

Scarry, Elaine, 102, 131
self-care, 133–134, 154–156, 161
Service, 1–5, 9, 22, 33, 54–59, 66, 72, 79, 93–95, 133–136, 160
Sevenhuijsen, Selma, 162
solace, 60, 87–88, 94–95
South Africa, 1, 3, 7, 49–50, 59, 72, 76, 80, 92–95, 104–106, 127, 130, 162–168
  Apartheid, 28
  C-section rates, 40, 64
  healthcare, 3
  history of birth, 28–34
  maternity care, 40
  medicalisation, 7–8, 22, 26, 28–32, 42, 46, 64, 151
  private sector, 1–2, 4–5, 26, 54, 140
  privilege, 36
  public sector, 2
  race, 10–11, 22, 25
  second tier health, 8
  third tier health, 8
stretch and sweep, 68, 173
studying up, 20
surges, 123

T

technologized birth, 33, 43
trust, 68–69, 76
  constructing, 79–81
  as a relation of care, 152–154
Tronto, Joan, 134, 145

U

universal feminine, 65, 71, 88–90, 93–95, 102, 115–117, 126–127

V

virtue, 124–125, 154
visibility, 21, 71, 88, 91–93
visible, 70–72, 90–93, 129,
visual, 15, 121
visualisation, 71, 106, 119, 124
voice, 71, 79, 91

W

women's work, 75, 81, 87, 115, 126–128

Y

Young, Iris, 144–145

www.ingramcontent.com/pod-product-compliance
Ingram Content Group UK Ltd.
Pitfield, Milton Keynes, MK11 3LW, UK
UKHW021839100926
8556IPUK00004B/432

9 781789 204353